Karl Otto
Greulich

# Micromanipulation by Light in Biology and Medicine

The Laser Microbeam and Optical Tweezers

Birkhäuser Verlag
Basel · Boston · Berlin

Author

Prof. Dr. Karl Otto Greulich
Institut für Molekulare Biotechnologie e.V.
Beutenbergstr. 11
D - 07708 Jena
Germany

Library of Congress Cataloging-in-Publication Data
Greulich, K. O. (Karl Otto), 1946–
    Micromanipulation by light in biology and medicine / K.O.
  Greulich.
  Includes bibliographical references and index.
    ISBN 0-8176-3873-3. -- ISBN 3-7643-3873-3
    1. Biology.  2. Medicine.  3. Micrurgy.  4. Light.  I. Title.
  QH307.2.G74  1999
  570'.28--dc21
                                          99-29317
                                          CIP


Deutsche Bibliothek Cataloging-in-Publication Data

**Greulich, Karl Otto**
Micromanipulation by light in biology and medicine : the laser
microbeam and optical tweezers / Karl Otto Greulich. – Basel ;
Boston ; Berlin : Birkhäuser, 1999

Cover Illustration: Götz Pilarczyk

© 1999 Birkhäuser Verlag, PO Box 133, CH-4010 Basel, Switzerland
Cover Design: Markus Etterich, Basel
Printed on acid-free paper produced from chlorine-free pulp. TCF ∞
Printed in Germany
ISBN 3-7643-3873-3
ISBN 0-8176-3873-3

9 8 7 6 5 4 3 2 1

# Table of contents

# Preface

There are probably few people who do not dream of the good old times, when doing science often meant fascination, excitement, even adventure. In our time, doing science involves often technology and, perhaps, even business. But there are still niches where curiosity and fascination have their place. The subject of this book, technological as its title may sound, is one of the fortunate examples. It will report on lasers generating the coldest places in the Universe, and on table top laser microtools which can produce a heat "inferno" as it prevails in the interior of the Sun, or simulate, for specific plant cells, microgravity of the space around our planet Earth. There will be some real surprises for the reader. The applications range from basic studies of the driving forces of cell division (and thus life) via genetic modification of cells (for example, for plant breeding) to medical applications such as blood cell analysis and finally *in vitro* fertilization.

What are these instruments: laser microbeams and optical tweezers? Both are lasers coupled with a fluorescence microscope. The laser microbeam uses a pulsed ultraviolet laser. Light is focused, as well as possible, in space and time, in order to obtain extremely high light intensities – high enough to generate, for a very short instant, extremely hot spots which can be used to cut, fuse or perforate biological material. Laser microbeams have evolved from microbeams with classical light sources which have been used in biology since the beginning of this century. Optical tweezers, on the other hand, use infrared lasers of moderate intensity and involve only little interaction with biological tissue. Their main purpose is to hold microscopic particles solely with the force of light or to measure microscopic forces with incredible precision. In some sense optical tweezers are an extended version of laser cooling of atoms and molecules.

Due to their different working principles, laser microbeams and optical tweezers so far have often been treated separately in the scientific literature. Reports on both microtools in combination are rare. Thus, this book is an attempt to bridge this gap and to use the synergy of both techniques. Interestingly, they are probably the only tools which allow one to work in the interiors of unopened objects – a truly exciting aspect.

This interdisciplinary book is intended to bridge a second gap: the gap between those who are new to the field (or who just want to learn more about it out of curiosity) and the specialists at the cutting edge of this field of research. Hopefully, the wide range of subjects presented will excite the interest of readers from many branches of science: physicists or chemists who want to learn how the dramatic effects of these tools can be used in biology, and biologists and physicians, who want to learn how the physical effects are generated. Certainly, the readers of this book will be of very different backgrounds. Therefore it is written on different levels. The main text should give the reader an overview. Details, hard stuff and data are presented in boxes, which the reader will wish or need to study in detail only if he or she wants a deeper understanding of the subject. For non-biologists, three sections called «intermezzos» are inserted which give some basic biological or biomedical information. Certainly these sections can not replace good textbooks, but they may give at least a foretaste of the biology and biomedicine described in subsequent chapters and sections. Finally, the information in the Appendix seeks to reduce the number of textbooks required by those who really want to build their own laser microbeam and optical tweezers.

I would like to thank all colleagues who have developed the techniques and have ingeniously used them to solve important questions of science. I hope that I have acknowledged their work properly by citing representative publications. Particularly I would like to thank Alla Margolina Litvin and Steve Block for numerous constructive critical comments.


Jena, 1 August 1998                                                    Karl Otto Greulich

# Introduction: The history of using light as a working tool

Certainly the earliest pioneers of optics realized that sunlight focused through a piece of curved glass can be used to perforate or slice thin pieces of wood or similar materials. Since then it has been known that light of a high power density can be used much like mechanical tools such as knives or scissors. At the beginning of this century, microscopists learned that a powerful conventional light source focused into a microscope could be used to manipulate biological objects. A conventional light source could be focused down to a spot size of a few micrometers. It was immediately clear that the "Strahlenstich", as it was called, was a tool for biologists. Probably the first work using highly focused light to manipulate biological material was that of S. Tschachotin (1912). Fig. 1 is a facsimile of the first page of Tschachotin' s paper.

> ### Die mikroskopische Strahlenstichmethode, eine Zelloperationsmethode.
> #### Von Dr. Sergeï Tschachotin.
> (Vorläufige Mitteilung.)
>
> (Aus der parasitologischen Abteilung [Vorstand: Prof. Dr. Th. v. Wasielewskij] des Instituts für Krebsforschung in Heidelberg, Direktor: Prof. Dr. V. Czerny, Exz., und aus dem pharmakologischen Institut der Universität Genua. Vorstand: Prof. Dr. A. Benedicenti.)
>
> Manche Gründe bewegen mich, einer Serie von Arbeiten, die noch nicht ganz abgeschlossen sind, diese vorläufige Mitteilung voranzuschicken.
>
> Den Anstoß zu den zu erwähnenden Untersuchungen gab die sich allmählich immer dringender einstellende Überzeugung, dass wir unsere erfolgreiche experimentelle Methodik, die in den letzten Jahrzehnten zu einem ungeahnten Fortschritt auf allen Gebieten der biologischen Forschung geführt hat, dimensional verfeinern und auf die kleinsten materiellen Einheiten des Lebens, auf die Zelle als Individuum, auszudehnen versuchen müssten.
>
> Wie wir beim Experiment in größerem Maßstabe praktisch-methodisch einen eingreifenden und einen registrierenden, beobachtenden Teil unterscheiden, so würde auch beim Mikroexperiment unser Augenmerk auf die Ausarbeitung erstens der Mikroläsions- und zweitens der Mikroobservationstechnik zu richten sein. Letztere kann bekanntlich subjektiv und objektiv (z. B. Mikrophotographie

**Fig. 1:** First page of Tschachotin' s paper on the «Strahlenstich» (which, today, could be translated as "microbeam").

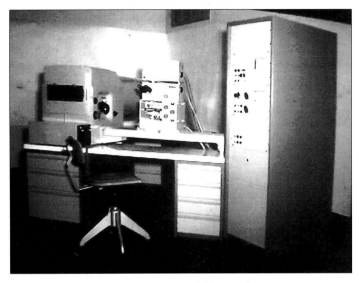

**Fig. 2:** *LMA 1, the first commercially available microbeam apparatus (Foto: V. Meinel and M. Ludwig, Jena).*

In spite of its age, the "Strahlenstich" is far from being old-fashioned. Whenever accuracies of a few micrometers and moderate power densities are sufficient the classical microbeam is as useful as the laser microbeam.

The latter, using a red ruby laser, became available in 1962 (Bessis et al., 1962), i.e. less than two years after the laser had been invented by Maiman (1960). In 1965, during an industry fair in Leipzig, Carl Zeiss, Jena, presented the LMA1 (laser microbeam analyzer) based on a ruby laser with microsecond pulses of a few millijoules each. Its spot size was approximately 2 micrometers.

In the early years, several groups had sporadically tried using the laser microbeam but then moved on to other topics. Since 1969 on, there has been a continuity in the use of laser microbeams. Michael Berns of the University of California at Irvine, published first papers on the use of laser microbeams in cell biology (Berns et al., 1969). He has continued this work with ever-increasing sophistication. A number of chapters of this book will be devoted to his studies.

Before the laser microbeam came of age, its application was split into two different directions. One direction was governed by work performed by Berns and his group (see, for example, Berns, 1974 or Berns et al., 1981). The second direction developed into molecular analysis: Laser ablation was combined with mass spectrometry and finally developed into laser mass analysis (LAMMA) and matrix assisted laser desorption (MALDI) (Hillenkamp et al. 1975). A variant of this is fluorescence recovery after photobleaching (FRAP, Peters, 1986). Here, fluorescent molecules on the surface of cells are bleached by highly focused laser pulses and the flow of molecules on the cell membrane is observed via fluorescence recovery. Today, the field of applications of laser microablation is so wide that not all aspects can be treated in a text the size of the present book. Therefore, reluctantly, its scope has to be limited, and LAMMA, MALDI and FRAP will not be covered in spite of the enormous impact they have.

The development of the optical tweezers is uniquely connected to the work of Arthur Ashkin from the AT&T Bell Labs in Holmdel, N J. (Ashkin, 1970). In the early seventies it was realized that the speed of an atom or a molecule can be reduced when a laser of a suitable color is directed into the direction of motion of the molecule. This phenomenon has been termed laser cooling since the speed of a molecule is related to its temperature, and it gained the 1997 Nobel prize in physics for S. Chu, W. Phillips and C. Cohen Tannoudji. Later it was shown that particles of the size of one micrometer, such as polystyrene beads, could also be manipulated by laser light. In that experiment, a focused laser was required and the particles were balanced on a focused laser beam, similar to a ping pong ball balanced on a jet of water. A significant step was the use of gradient forces which, in contrast to light pressure, pull dielectric particles into the focus of a laser, i.e. they can also be moved against the direction light propagation. The set up for such an experiment was named "single beam optical trap" or "optical tweezers" (Ashkin et al., 1986). Even today, both expressions are used in the scientific community and will be used interchangeably throughout this book.

Until 1987 the single beam gradient trap was used successfully only with non-living material. Then, Ashkin's group published two papers changing the field dramatically. The breakthrough for the use of the optical trap in biology came when viruses and bacteria were first trapped with a green argon ion laser (Ashkin and Dziedzic, 1987) and subsequently an infrared NdYAG laser was used for manipulation of whole cells (Ashkin et al., 1987). This change from green to infrared was an important step since infrared light with a wavelength of about one micrometer is only weakly absorbed by biological material. Fragile mammalian cells survived this laser treatment. This was the beginning of optical trapping in cell biology. The end of the decade was the time of pioneers in optical trapping, most notably among them were the groups of Todor Buican (Buican 1987) and Steven Block (Block 1989) and of course, Arthur Ashkin.

In 1989 the microbeam field and the optical trapping field were merged by the first combination of laser microbeams and optical tweezers (Greulich et al., 1989, Greulich et al 1990). From then on complete micromanipulation by light was possible with one single piece of equipment. The last decade of this millenium is now witnessing a dramatic expansion of the field. Micromanipulation by light may be on the way to becoming a standard tool for many fields of science.

**Box 1: Milestones in the development of laser microbeams and optical tweezers**

| | |
|---|---|
| 1912 | S. Tschachotin publishes the first work on the microbeam using a thermal light source |
| 1917 | A. Einstein develops the theoretical foundations of lasers |
| 1961 | M. Maiman presents the first laser |
| 1962 | Bessis present the first laser microbeam |
| 1969 | Berns develops microbeams into a standard tool for many fields of biology |
| 1968/70 | Letokhov and Ashkin publish the principles of using light pressure to manipulate atoms, molecules and microscopic particles |
| 1986 | The single beam gradient trap (optical tweezers ) |
| 1987 | Ashkin's papers on the use of *infrared* gradient traps with living objects |
| 1989 | First quantitative force measurements with optical tweezers by the groups of Ashkin and Block |
| 1989 | Combination of the laser microbeam and the optical tweezers |
| 1989–now | Complete micromanipulation by light |
| 1997 | Physics Nobel Prize for cooling atoms and molecules by light |

## Selected literature

A. Ashkin (1970) Acceleration and trapping of particles by radiation pressure. Phys. Rev. Lett. 24: 156–159.

A. Ashkin, J.M. Dziedzic, J.E. Bjorkholm, S. Chu (1986) Observation of a single beam gradient trap for dielectric particles. Optics Letters 11, 288–290.

A. Ashkin, J.M. Dziedzic (1987) Optical trapping and manipulation of viruses and bacteria. Science 235, 1517–20.

A. Ashkin, A., J.M. Dziedzic, T. Yamane (1987) Optical trapping and manipulation of single cells using infrared laser beams. Nature 330, 769–771.

T.N. Buican, M.J. Smith, H.A. Crissmann, G.C. Salzmann, C.C. Stewart, J.C. Martin (1987) Automated single cell manipulation and sorting by light trapping. Appl. Opt. 26, 5311–5316.

M.W. Berns (1974) Prentice Hall Series on Biological Techniques, Englewood Cliffs, New Jersey. Biological microirradiation.

M.W. Berns, D.E. Rounds, R.S. Olson (1969) Effects of laser microirradiation on chromosomes. Exp. Cell. Res. 56, 292–298.

M.W. Berns, J. Aist, J. Edwards, K. Strahs, J. Girton, P McNeill, J.B. Rattner, M. Kitzes, M. Hammer-Wilson, L.H. Liaw, A. Siemens, M. Koonce, S. Peterson, S. Brenner, J. Burt, R. Walter, P.J. Bryant, D van Dyk, J. Coulombe, T. Cahill, G.S. Berns (1981) Laser microsurgery in cell and developmental biology. Science 213, 505–513.

M. Bessis, F. Gires, G. Mayer, G. Nomarski (1962) Irradiation des organites cellulaires a l'aide d'un laser a rubis (Irradiation of cellular organisms with a ruby laser) C.R. Acad. Sci. 255, 1010–1012.

S.M. Block, D.F. Blair, H.C. Berg. (1989) Compliance of bacterial flagella measured with optical tweezers. Nature 338, 514–18.

K.O Greulich, U. Bauder, S. Monajembashi, N. Ponelies, S. Seeger, J. Wolfrum (1989) UV Laser Mikrostrahl und optische Pinzette (UV laser microbeam and optical tweezers) Labor Praxis/Labor 2000, 36–42.

K.O. Greulich, S. Monajembashi, S. Seeger, J. Wolfrum 1990 Cytometry, Application of optical trapping in molecular genetics, immunology and cell fusion. Suppl.4, 18 (83).

F. Hillenkamp, E. Unsöld, R. Kaufmann, R. Nitsche (1975) Laser microprobe mass analysis of organic materials. Nature 256, 119–120.

V.S. Lethokhov (1968) Toward laser cooling of molecular motion. Pis'ma Zh. Exp.

Theor. Fiz 7, 348, see also: 1995 Ber. Bunsenges. Phys. Chem 95. 3, 498–503.

T. Maiman (1960) Stimulated optical radiation in ruby masers. Nature 187, 493–494.

R. Peters (1986) Fluorescence microphotolysis to measure nucleocytoplasmic transport and intracellular mobility. Bioch. Bioph. Acta 864, 305–359.

S. Tschachotin (1912) Die mikroskopische Strahlenstichmethode, eine Zelloperationsmethode. (The microbeam, a cell operation method) Biol. Zentralbl. 32, 623–630.

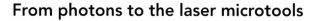

# 1 From photons to the laser microtools

## 1.1 Light

In everyday life we perceive light as a gentle physical entity. Using light to destroy or to transport objects – sometimes even in the interior of a closed room – appears to be a matter of science fiction. Surprisingly, it is science, almost lab routine – at least in the world of microscopy. Light can be used as a quasi-mechanical working tool.

In this first chapter you will learn that light can do more than just illuminate things. You will find out why light transmits not only heat (energy) but also exerts pressure and force.

In the chapters thereafter you will get a glimpse of how lasers produce a peculiar light – light which can be used to work at a distance, without any direct mechanical contact. When combined with a microscope, the light of a comparably small desktop laser can be focused to such high intensities that it will produce temperatures as they prevail in the interior of the Sun (laser microbeams) and that objects can be moved by some mysterious, at first glance, force (optical tweezers) – even through a wall which you could hardly penetrate with a mechanical tool.

### 1.1.1 Light is a special form of electromagnetic radiation

The proof that light is electromagnetic radiation is one of the most dramatic feats of physics. Historically, it took decades of research on electricity and magnetism, before James Clerk Maxwell (1873) could unify a plethora of different physical laws and created a system of four equations from which, in principle, all laws of electricity and magnetism can be derived. Using a special combination of these Maxwell equations one finally ends up with an equation which is only satisfied for a physical entity which has wave properties. And not only that! The equation can be solved correctly only when these waves travel exactly with the velocity of light.

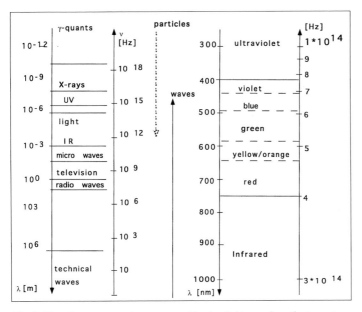

**Fig. 3:** *The electromagnetic spectrum: On the right wavelengths in meters and frequencies in Hz of the whole range from γ-quants to technical waves are shown. The left gives the range of the visible spectrum, with wavelengths in nanometers. In the center the ranges are indicated where we perceive electromagnetic radiation as waves or as particles.*

These are the electromagnetic waves. Light is a special form of the much wider spectrum of electromagnetic waves (radiowaves, microwaves, X-rays). Our eyes "measure" the wavelength of light via its color. Wavelengths of visible light range from 0.4 micrometers (blue) to 0.8 micrometers (red). Wavelengths below 0.4 μm are invisible (ultraviolet). For example, UV light responsible for suntan has a wavelength between 0.35 and 0.4 μm. Wavelengths above 0.8 μm are also invisible. Here the regime of (near) infrared radiation begins. For comparison, high quality mechanical workpieces can have an accuracy of that size and thin plastic or aluminum foils may also be a few wavelengths thick. Fig. 3 gives an overview over the whole spectrum of electromagnetic waves.

Since wavelengths of known electromagnetic waves range from femtometers ($10^{-15}$ m, cosmic rays) to kilometers (long radio waves) visible light represents in fact only a marginal part of the electromagnetic spectrum. Of the 18 orders of magnitude which are covered by electromagnetic radiation known so far, visible light covers less than one order of magnitude. If one were to represent all these wavelengths on a linear scale with the length of Earth's equator, the visible spectrum of light would cover 16 cm.

## 1.1.2 The energy carried by light

A look at a radio receiver shows, quite often, that the positions of radio stations are given in kilohertz or megahertz as well as in meters or centimeters. Obviously, frequency $\nu$ and wavelength $\lambda$ are somehow equivalent. In fact, their product, a velocity, is always the same, whether it is calculated for X-rays, ultraviolet or visible light, microwaves or radio waves. It is

$$c = \lambda \cdot \nu, \quad (1)$$

and c is always the velocity of light, in vacuum (and approximately also in air)

$$c = 2.9979 \cdot 10^8 \text{ m/sec.} \quad (2)$$

For most purposes one can write $c = 3 \cdot 10^{10}$ cm/sec or $3 \cdot 10^8$ m/sec. The velocity can be much smaller in matter; for example by a factor of 2.7 in diamond. If you want to learn more about this aspect, turn to the Appendix for details.

There is no upper limit for the amount of energy which a beam of light can exchange with matter. However, it was one of the big milestones of science when it was realized that there is a minimum portion (quantum) of energy which can be exchanged. It is related to the frequency of the light wave

$$E = h \cdot \nu \quad (3)$$

where h (the Planck constant) is $6.6 \cdot 10^{-27}$ gcm$^2$/s. Combining Equations 1 and 3 one obtains
$$E = h \cdot c / \lambda. \quad (4)$$

It is this energy which is used in industrial processes to cut or weld slabs of steel or plastics by lasers. We will finally use this energy in the laser microbeam. Surely, in order to cut or weld metal slabs, one needs very large numbers of these light quanta. In Boxes 2 and 3 it is shown how these numbers can be calculated and how they are related to energy quantities such as the "Calorie" or the "Joule", or to power quantities such as the "Watt".

## Box 2: Units of force, energy and power

### Force

In everyday life we say that an object weighs X grams. This is not totally correct . In the strict language of physics the gram defines the mass, but only indirectly the weight. A mass of 1kg will remain 1 kg on the surface of the Earth and in space. The weight depends on gravity and is expressed as the force which is acting on an object. The formula to calculate this is

$$F = m \cdot g,$$

where g is the gravitational acceleration (approx. $10 \text{ ms}^{-2}$). At the surface of the Earth a mass of 1 kg feels a force of 1 kg ms$^{-2}$ or 1 kilopond. This is , in a different system of physical units, 10 newtons. Since in space the gravitational acceleration g is almost zero, objects in space are weightless. Typical forces which will be exerted by optical tweezers are in the nanonewton ($10^{-9}$ newton) range or below.

### Energy

Energy may be defined in many different ways. One definition is

$$1 \text{ Joule} = 1 \text{ newton·meter (Nm)}$$

Physically this means that, when an object is moved along a distance of 1 meter with a force of one newton (for example, against friction) , an energy of 1 Joule is required. The Joule can be correlated with the certainly best known energy quantity:

$$1 \text{ Joule} = 0.2421 \text{ calories} \quad \text{or} \quad 1 \text{ calorie} = 4.13 \text{ Joule.}$$

One calorie heats one gram of water by one degree. A man needs a few million calories or a few thousand kilocalories per day, i.e. the amount of energy which would be sufficient to heat 100 kg of water by 10°C.

### Power

The power is defined as energy per time.

$$1 \text{ Watt} = 1 \text{ Joule per second.}$$

Light bulbs have to be powered with some tens of Watts, cars with some tens (or more) of Kilowatts. For more details see Box 12 in Section 2.1.

### Intensity

Intensity (or power density) is the power per area (Watt per cm$^2$).

## Box 3: The number of light quanta contained in a pulse of a given energy

For a number of applications it is useful to have a relationship between the energy of a light quantum and macroscopic energies. Here you can learn how such relationships are calculated in detail:

The product $h \cdot c$ in Equation 4 is

$$h \cdot c = (6.6 \cdot 10^{-27} \text{ g} \cdot \text{cm}^2/\text{s}) \cdot (3 \cdot 10^{10} \text{ cm/s})$$

$$h \cdot c = 19.8 \cdot 10^{-17} \text{ g} \cdot \text{cm}^3/\text{s}^2.$$

For a quantum of green light (500 nm) the energy can be calculated as

$$E = 19.8 \cdot 10^{-17} \text{ g} \cdot \text{cm}^3 \cdot \text{s}^{-2}/500 \cdot 10^{-7} \text{ cm}$$

$$E = 3.96 \cdot 10^{-12} \text{ g} \cdot \text{cm}^2/\text{s}^2.$$

Since

$$10^7 \text{ g} \cdot \text{cm}^2/\text{s} = 1 \text{ Nm} = 1 \text{ J}.$$

the energy of a green light quantum is

$$E = 3.96 \cdot 10^{-19} \text{ J}$$

The reciprocal of this gives the number of quanta required to add up to 1 Joule:

$$2.5 \cdot 10^{18} \text{ green light quanta per Joule}$$

In order to calculate how many quanta of other wavelengths (for example 337 nm) are needed to make 1 Joule, one just has to multiply it with the wavelength ratio (for example 337/500). Thus 1 J corresponds to $1.7 \cdot 10^{18}$ quanta of UV light at 337 nm wavelength.

A mean-sized laser may provide a power of 1 W. As we have seen above, this corresponds to $2.5 \cdot 10^{18}$ of green light quanta per second, i.e. a relativistic mass of the order of 10 femtograms (1 fg=$10^{-15}$g) is flowing per second. For comparison the Sun radiates $3.8 \cdot 10^{26}$ W and thus its mass decreases by approx. 4.5 million tons per second .

### 1.1.3 Photons and their social behavior

Albert Einstein, although one of the fathers of the photon concept, complained in 1951 about his own limited knowledge of photons: "Heute glaubt zwar jeder Lump, er wisse es, aber er täuscht sich" ["Nowadays every fool thinks he knows it, but he is wrong."].

Surprisingly, not too much has changed since then. Nobody can say how large a photon is. Does the photon have the size of the wavelength? Or is it a point-like particle which jitters so much through the world that we think it should have the size of the wavelength? Or is it something in-between? Quantum mechanics by no means gives any information on the shape of such a portion of energy and therefore the picture of the photon as being, strictly, a particle is misleading. Particularly, it is not possible to conclude that the photon is a point-like particle. The photon is an energy quantum which can be exchanged during interaction of light with matter and whose energy can be calculated by Equation 3 or 4 – that's all! We should keep this in mind, but we should not worry too much about it. In the following we will use the terms "photon" and "quantum" almost interchangeably.

In a group of photons traveling through space it is not possible to assign a number to one particular photon and to expect to find it later again, after the group has traveled a distance through space. Photons belong to a special class of elementary particles; they are "bosons". Unlike their counterparts, the fermions (for example, electrons) which tend to avoid the company of a second fermion, bosons seek the company of others. That's the reason why the Bose-Einstein condensation is possible, the experimental verification of which has recently excited so many physicists. If one photon meets a second one, both tend to travel together, and they tend to gather as many companions as possible. In more professional terminology:

*photons as bosons tend to occur in the same quantum state.*

It is this property which allows us to concentrate large numbers of photons in space and in time to finally use light as a working tool, and it is this property which makes the laser work and finally allows us to generate extremely high light intensities in the laser microbeam and to some extent in optical tweezers.

## 1.1.4 The (relativistic) mass of a photon

The photon is a massless particle. To be precise, one should say that a photon at rest, i.e. at speed zero, has no mass. In fact the formal photon mass at rest is zero. But photons at rest do not exist. Photons always travel. In vacuum, they travel always with the speed of light $c=3\cdot10^8$ m/sec, (see section 1.1.1) And there is something strange with objects travelling with a speed close or equal to c. Their mass increases with increasing speed. One important equation from Einstein's theory of relativity allows us to calculate the mass m at a speed v from the mass at rest, $m_o$:

$$m = m_o/\sqrt{(1-v^2/c^2)}. \quad (5)$$

This is correct for any object, also for your own mass. But even for astronauts in the fastest known space crafts the difference between their rest mass $m_o$ and their relativistic mass m cannot be measured. At 10% of the speed of light, which for macroscopic objects is far from any technical reality, the mass increases only by one half percent. However, when the speed v of an object approaches c, the term $v^2/c^2$ approaches 1 and consequently the square root in the denominator of Equation 5 goes to zero. Thus the mass of a particle traveling close to the speed of light increases dramatically. That is the reason why one needs kilometer-sized accelerators to speed up electrons (which at speed zero are really light weights) to velocities close to c. There is one exception: when the formal mass $m_o$ is zero, as is the case for the photon, the whole expression becomes 0/0. This is not equal to 1, as one might expect. Mathematical rules say that this ratio has to be carefully calculated by alternative means.

This alternative approach uses the probably best known formula of physics

$$E = m\cdot c^2 \quad (6)$$

which implies that energy is always correlated with a mass m, irrespective of any strictly particle-like structure. Equation 4 can be rearranged and combined with Equation 6.

$$m = E/c^2 = (h/\lambda)\cdot c \quad (7)$$

and one can calculate, for example, that a green light quantum (with a wavelength of 500 nm) carries a relativistic mass of $4 \cdot 10^{-33}$ g, which is about 1:225000 of the mass of an electron at rest ($9 \cdot 10^{-28}$ g).

## 1.1.5 Light pressure: Where does it come from?

In this chapter you will learn why light falling onto an object exerts pressure and force on this object and thus you get a first glimpse of the working principle of laser cooling and of optical tweezers. For this we need another physical quantity: the translational momentum T. This is just the product of the photon's mass and its speed, for a photon:

$$T = m \cdot c. \quad (8)$$

By replacing the mass m using Equation 6 one immediately obtains

$$T = E/c \quad (9)$$

When an object changes its speed, and thus its momentum T, a force will be involved. For example, when you use brakes on your car, reducing speed from 20 mph to zero within five sec, a moderate force is acting. If you, involuntarily, do the same within a tenth of this time, in 0.5 sec, e.g. by driving your car against an obstacle, then a tenfold force will act.

Obviously the force is related to the change in momentum per time. This can be expressed as

$$F = T/t. \quad (10)$$

More precisely, one has to write the "differentials", $P = dT/dt$ , but this is not too important for the following calculation.
When T is replaced by E/c (see Equation 9) one obtains

$$F = E/(c \cdot t). \quad (11)$$

Since the energy per time is defined as the power W (= E/t), one ends up with an extremely simple equation for the calculation of forces exerted by light:

$$F = W/c. \quad (12)$$

In order to calculate the light pressure P, one has to divide the whole equation by the cross-section area S (since P is defined as F/S). On the right side of the equation, we then end up with an expression W/S , i.e. power per area. This is the power density or intensity of light I. Using this quantity, the equation for light pressure adopts the same form as the force equation:

$$P = I/c. \quad (13)$$

Equations 12 and 13 are correct in vacuum. In a solvent with refractive index $n_1$ (an optical material constant) they must be corrected via multiplying by the latter. Thus the equations for the force and the pressure exerted by light falling onto an object become

$$F = n_1 \cdot W/c \quad (14)$$

and

$$P = n_1 \cdot I/c \quad (15)$$

where $n_1$ is the refractive index of the medium (in biological experiments often water with $n_1 = 1.3345$).

## 1.1.6 Cooling of atoms and molecules by light: What optical tweezers have in common with the coldest place in the Universe

Light forces act on any particle – charged, magnetic or neutral. Already around 1970 it was suggested to exploit this effect for the trapping of atoms and other neutral particles (Letokhov 1968, Ashkin 1970). The 1997 Physics Nobel Prize winners S. Chu, W.D. Phillips and C. Cohen Tannoudji have developed these ideas into practical applications, particularly into cooling of neutral atoms and molecules by light. Motion is related to temperature. For example, thermal motion is fast for hot objects and slow for cold objects. Thus, reducing an atom's or a molecule's speed is equivalent to cooling it.

Extremely small thermal motions can be generated when momentum transfer (see Equations 8-10) during absorption is exploited. By absorption, light moving at $3 \cdot 10^{10}$

cm/sec is braked to the speed of the absorbing atom or molecule, transfers its momentum and thus changes the speed of the latter. It can either brake or accelerate an atom or molecule: without a further trick, this process is not suitable for cooling.

Here a process is important which most readers probably know from sound. When a police car approaches you, its horn has a relatively high tone, corresponding to a high frequency or short wavelength. After it has passed you, the sound becomes lower, corresponding to a longer wavelength. This is called the "Doppler effect". In some sense the sound of the police car siren in the two situations has different apparent wavelengths. By a similar effect, an atom traveling against the direction of a light beam absorbs light with a little bit shorter wavelength than it would absorb at zero speed. When such light with a slightly too short wavelength is used for the cooling of atoms, only such atoms are reduced in speed which are running against the beam, but others are not affected. In other words: atoms are either not affected at all or they are cooled down. After a while, all atoms or molecules are cooled down. The process has been termed "Doppler cooling."

Doppler cooling allows the generation of temperatures as low as 0.2 micro-Kelvin when the relatively heavy cesium atoms are used. With low weight helium atoms temperatures of 23 micro-Kelvin can be generated, corresponding to a speed of 9.2 cm per sec for each single helium atom. The reason for this limitation is that every atom or molecule which has absorbed light will finally re-emit it (see, for example, section 1.2). This emission causes a recoil and will speed up the atom or molecule again.

With some atoms such as a special variant of helium (1s2s3S-helium) a further trick allows even lower temperatures. One can take care that atoms which are already slow can be transferred into a dark state where they do not re-emit light within a limited time span. Using this "sub-recoil cooling", helium atoms have been cooled down to 4 micro-Kelvins, corresponding to a speed of 2 cm per sec. Four micro-Kelvins is really cold – only four millionths of a degree away from the coldest temperature theoretically possible. The temperature of the Universe is higher. Thus, the combination of the techniques described above is responsible for the fact that the coldest place in the Universe is not somewhere far away in deep space but in a laboratory on this planet Earth. What does all that have to do with optical tweezers? Doppler cooling and sub-recoil cooling represent one branch of sophisticated developments of the original ideas of using light to manipulate objects. They will probably not find a lot of applications in biology and biomedicine, simply since such tremendous accuracies are probably not needed in studies on biological macromolecules, cells or tissues. A second branch of application is represented by optical tweezers. They work particularly well at temperatures where living objects are active. Under suitable conditions optical tweezers do not affect viability. This will be the subject of many chapters throughout this book.

## Summary and outlook

We have learned that light is a carrier of energy and of momentum. We can use this property to generate the coldest spots in the Universe. In turn, if we could manage to send light of sufficient intensity in a given direction we would be able to transmit energy and exert force at a distance – just as is described in many science fiction stories. What we need is a suitable light source. Such a source is available: the laser.

## Selected literature

A. Ashkin (1970) Acceleration and trapping of particles by radiation pressure. Phys. Rev. Lett. 24, 156–59.

S. Chu (1992) Laser trapping of neutral particles. Scientific American 2, 71–76.

J. Lawall, S. Kulin, B. Saubamea, N. Bigelow, M. Leduc, C. Cohen-Tannoudji (1995) Three-dimensional laser cooling of helium beyond the single-photon recoil limit. Phys. Rev. Lett. 75, 4194–4197.

V.S. Lethokhov (1968) Toward laser cooling of molecular motion. Pis'ma Zh. Exp. Theor. Fiz 7, 348, see also: (1995) Ber. Bunsenges. Phys. Chem 95. 3, 498–503.

W.D. Phillips, HJ. Metcalf (1987) Cooling and trapping atoms. Scientific American 1, 36–42.

# 1.2 Lasers: sources of peculiar light

Have you ever held a laser pointer in your hands? Have you felt the fascination when you realized that the spot generated does not increase, even when you direct it onto an object far in front of you? If not, just try it.

When the laser, theoretically envisioned already by Albert Einstein, was invented (Maiman, 1960) it was ridiculed as a "a solution in search of a problem". In other words, the laser was thought of as a useless invention. Today, almost everybody owns a laser – in a CD player, in a computer printer or photocopier – or has at least made use of it, for example by listening to a friend' s CD or perhaps in medical analysis or therapy.

The reason for its success is that the laser is really a peculiar source of light – and that the light generated by lasers is peculiar.

### 1.2.1 Laser light: Spectral purity, coherence and divergence

Fig. 4 shows the specific features of laser light as compared to the light of a standard bulb.

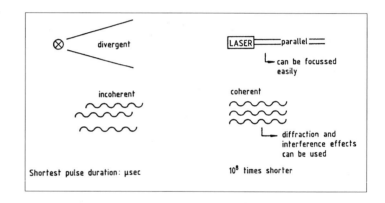

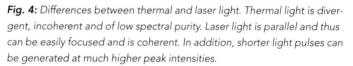

**Fig. 4:** *Differences between thermal and laser light. Thermal light is divergent, incoherent and of low spectral purity. Laser light is parallel and thus can be easily focused and is coherent. In addition, shorter light pulses can be generated at much higher peak intensities.*

Three features can be distinguished:
1. The light of a bulb is emitted in all directions of space while the laser light is almost parallel. One says that the laser has a small divergence. A small divergence is very important for laser microtools since there one will finally attempt to focus light to the theoretical (diffraction) limit. The divergence angle is the fraction of the surface area of a unit sphere (i.e. a sphere with radius 1 cm) which is illuminated by a light source located in its center. Since the surface of a sphere is generally $4\pi r^2$ and that of a unit sphere is $4\pi$, a standard bulb which illuminates all parts of the sphere has a divergence of $4\pi$. Good lasers, in turn, have divergences as low as $10^{-8}$, i.e. they would illuminate an area of a few mm diameter on a sphere with radius 1 cm. In conclusion

*the divergence of lasers may be nine orders of magnitude smaller than
the divergence of classical light sources.*

2.  A second property of laser light is its high spectral purity. For practically all purposes of laser micromanipulation by light the laser light consists of virtually one single wavelength. Quantitatively this is expressed as bandwidth of frequencies $\Delta v$, where $c = \lambda \cdot v$ (Eq.1) is used to convert wavelengths into frequencies. Even with the cheapest lasers it is no problem to generate light in which the different wavelengths vary by less than one tenth of a nanometer. Only spectroscopists need even better-defined laser light. Their efforts have shown that the wavelength purity can exceed the nanometer accuracy by many orders of magnitude.

*Laser light consists of only one wavelength while classical sources even
after optical filtering, provide a mixture of wavelengths.*

3.  Lasers produce very long wave trains. They have a large "coherence length". This is the length within which the front of the wavetrain is correlated with the end by one single sinus function (see also Box A8 in Appendix A4.1).

*Coherence lengths of lasers are up to 14 orders of magnitude larger
than those of classical light.*

The coherence length $l_{coh}$ and the spectral purity, expressed as the bandwidth of frequencies, $\Delta v$ which are present in the light are correlated with each other by a basic law of quantum optics

$$l_{coh} = c/\Delta v. \quad (16)$$

When $\Delta v$ is small, i.e. when the light has a high spectral purity, the coherence length becomes large. The coherence length is a measure of the quality of the laser light. In Box 4 coherence lengths for a number of light sources are listed.

**Box 4: Coherence length and divergence of different light sources**

| Light source | Coherence length | Divergence |
|---|---|---|
| The Sun | 0.6 µm | $4\pi$ |
| Best classical source | 30 cm | $4\pi$ |
| Ruby and Neodym YAG | 10 m | $10^{-6}$ |
| He/Ne Laser | 3 m | $10^{-8}$ |
| He/Ne stabilized | 400000 km | $10^{-9}$ |
| Argon ion laser | 300 m | $10^{-8}$ |

## 1.2.2 Principles of lasing

A laser, as does any light source, uses the fact that atoms or molecules can be excited by several types of energy and can re-emit part of that energy as light. This is true of classical (thermal) light bulbs as well as lasers.

There are two types of emission. One is spontaneous, i.e. after some time of being excited the atom emits light into an arbitrary direction of space. Light bulbs using this type of emission will generate light with high divergence. Lasers use a different type of emission, first detected by Albert Einstein. When an excited atom or molecule is hit by light with the same wavelength as it would emit spontaneously, it is stimulated to emit its photon earlier than it would without being stimulated. And, since it is a boson (see section 1.1.3 on the social behaviour of photons) it will join the stimulating wave of light and travel in the same direction. In a long cylinder filled with excited atoms or molecules, this will happen again and again. Light traveling not parallel to the cylinder axis will finally hit the side walls of the cylinder and will be absorbed. But light traveling (almost) parallel will be amplified. We have **L**ight **A**mplification by **S**timulated **E**mission of **R**adiation. The first letters have been used to abbreviate the description of this physical process, and the word **LASER** has now become an accepted word in everyday language and even the verb "to lase" can now be found in dictionaries.

One can optically increase the length of the cylinder by attaching mirrors to the front end of it. Then the light travels many times up and down the cylinder. One of the mirrors reflects 100% of the impinging light, the other is partly transparent. Part of the light is reflected and goes through additional cycles of amplification. The other part leaves the laser as a highly parallel beam with only very small divergence.

Placing a computer-operated mirror in the path of this beam generates the beautiful light shows known from discotheques. Directing it on a car and measuring the light reflected from the car's metal surface allows one to measure velocity. Coupling the beam with a microscope is the first step toward building microbeams and optical tweezers.

### 1.2.3 Inversion, three and four energy-state lasers

Sections 1.2.3 through 1.2.6 will show you that only special types of atoms or molecules are suited as laser media, that some special physical conditions are required to generate laser light and that you may use many different types of energy sources in order to "pump" lasers. You will also learn that lasers provide very special intensity patterns (modes) and that it is possible, with the help of crystals, to change the color of laser light by frequency doubling, tripling etc.

Excited atoms are like spanned springs with aging spanning mechanisms. They usually relax spontaneously within a time period of the order of 10 ns. Stimulated emission can only occur before a spontaneous decay. In order to improve that process a large number of excited atoms (or, to use our mechanical image, spanned springs) must accumulate before they emit spontaneously. Actually, the number of atoms $n_b$ in the excited state must be larger than the number $n_a$ of atoms in the the ground state. This situation is called "inversion". A physicochemical law (the Boltzmann law) prohibits such an inversion since, strictly speaking, this would entail negative absolute temperatures. In principle, the Boltzmann law says that in thermal equilibrium the number of atoms or molecules in a state of given energy decreases exponentially with increasing energy. Since an excited state has, by definition, a higher energy level than the ground state, the number of atoms or molecules in this state is smaller than in the ground state, i.e. there is no chance for inversion.

The trick is to use atoms or molecules which have at least a third energy state (see also Appendix A5). The third state (which we will call the "upper lasing state") has a lifetime of a factor of 100 or more longer than the excited state. A few percent of the excited atoms or molecules do not emit the light spontaneously by a transition into the ground state but convert it into the long-living third state by a process called intersystem crossing. This process liberates the system from the constraints imposed by the Boltzmann law. The number $n_c$ of atoms in the upper lasing state increases until it is larger than the number $n_a$ of atoms in the ground state, i.e. until inversion occurs. To some extent the situation is comparable to a river which is partly bypassed by a channel with barriers. In spite of the fact that only a small amount of water flows through the channel, there is a last barrier at its end, where energy can be gained, for example in a small power station. This last barrier corresponds to the laser transition.

The ruby laser, the first laser ever constructed, and the nitrogen laser, which will be used for the microbeams, are examples of three-state lasers. They have disadvantages: In the three-state system one has no control over the ground state. Such control is possible in a four-state system, as it is realized in Neodymium (Nd) lasers, among them the NdYAG laser which is used for optical tweezers (Fig. 5).

In Fig. 5 it becomes obvious that excitation and the laser transition are uncoupled from each other. What is now the advantage of a fourth state, which we will call the "lower lasing state"? It has a very short lifetime. Whenever it is populated by an emisson from the upper lasing state, it will immediately emit its energy and transit into the ground state. Therefore, the lower lasing state is virtually depopulated; $n_d$ is almost zero. Inversion is already achieved when only a few atoms are in the upper lasing state. In other words, it is easy to obtain inversion in this pair of states.

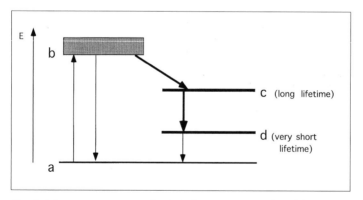

**Fig. 5:** *A four-state system as a basis for lasing. Due to its long lifetime the state c becomes populated while the short-living state d, is always depopulated. For details see text.*

## 1.2.4 Pumping: The primary energy source for lasers

Stimulated emission can continue only as long as inversion exists. Then the inversion has to be regenerated. This can be done by classical light with a wavelength approximately in the correct range, for example, in flash lamp pumped lasers. Often, an electric gas discharge or sometimes just simple heating or a suitable chemical reaction is sufficient to excite this process. It may sound strange that even lasers are used to pump this excitation. For example, the transition between the gound state and the excited state may happen to fit the working wavelength of a cheap laser, while the transition between the upper and the lower lasing states generates a wavelength which can only be accomplished by expensive lasers. In such a case, pumping by a laser is a very economic way to generate the otherwise "expensive" light. The NdYAG laser which is quite often used for optical tweezers is a very good example: the flash lamp pumped versions are increasingly being replaced by diode laser pumped versions. The latter are much smaller in size, and thus better suitable to be used together with a microscope. In addition, they convert a much higher percentage of electrical energy into laser light since they produce much less useless heat.

For regeneration of the inversion one may imagine that the laser works in two phases. First, the inversion is generated by excitation from the gound state to the excited state. Subsequently, the emission will be stimulated. Occasionally this is achieved by switching the semi-transparent mirror between fully reflecting (during regeneration of inversion) to partly transparent (in order to couple the light out) Such a strategy results in a Q-switched (Q stands for the reflection quality of the mirror) pulsed laser. There are additional ways to get a pulsed laser, such as by "mode locking", but this will not be discussed here.

At least in some laser media, it is also possible to regenerate the inversion simultaneously with the simulated emission. Since the stimulation occurs at a wavelength other than the pumping laser transition, the two processes do not interfere. One achieves some equilibrium between pumping and lasing, as in the river example above, where a continuous flow of water fuels the channel and power can still be gained at the last barrier. By such a strategy, a continuously working laser is possible, provided that a few other conditions are met. These will be described in the next section.

## 1.2.5 Laser resonators and laser modes (see also Appendix A4.4)

The two mirrors at the end of the lasing cylinder form a cavity. When waves are confined in cavities, those wavelengths which perfectly fit have an advantage and are thus particularly amplified, while other wavelengths are attenuated. A comparison with a string of a violin is appropriate: in principle such a string can generate a number of different tones. By pressing a finger on a selected point on the string one defines its active length. The tone with the acoustic wavelength which optimally fits on the length of this section of the string will be amplified while other tones will be suppressed. Therefore, a very pure tone will be generated. In a laser cavity the situation is comparable: when the distance between the two mirrors is exactly a multiple integer of the half wavelength of the laser transition (i.e. to the energy difference between upper and lower lasing state), then a standing wave is built up in the laser cavity. Fig. 6 shows how this results in amplification of one specific wavelength.

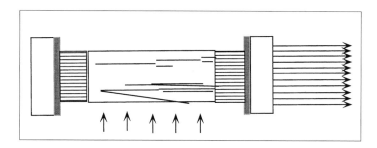

**Fig. 6:** *Process of light amplification in a laser. The cylindrical laser medium is pumped via the large surface area of the cylinder. Amplification occurs along the optical axis between the mirrors at the front ends. Some stimulated waves do not reach the mirrors and are lost; others are amplified several times.*

The length of a typical laser resonator is measured in cm while the wavelength of light is half a micron; i.e., several ten thousand wavelengths fit into a laser cavity. At such a large number it is possible that other wavelengths may also happen to fit well between the two mirrors. This is not a serious problem with wavelengths which are not generated at all by the stimulated emission. However, since the energy difference between the upper and lower lasing state varies slightly from atom to atom (the energy states are not ideally narrow) they emit bands of wavelengths (though very narrow ones). Any wavelength of this band which fits into the laser cavity will be amplified – these are the different longitudinal modes of a laser. For use in laser micromanipulation by light this fact is irrelevant, since the different wavelengths are close enough to each other to be regarded as one spectrally pure line. For the spectroscopist, who needs much higher wavelength resolution, the different longitudinal laser modes may be a problem and he has to take measures accordingly.

More relevant are the transversal modes: The medium, often a gas, has to be held in a cylinder of a specified diameter. The cylinder walls represent a second type of spatial limitation of the laser wave, now not in the direction of light propagation but perpendicular to it. In a way quite similar as described for the longitudinal waves, this fact causes transversal modes (TEMs, tranversal electromagnetic modes). These modes generate interesting patterns: their cross section may, for example, be a ring (doughnut) or a well-ordered system of points. They are comparable to the vibration modes of a drumhead. TEMs are designated by two indices which represent the class of mathematical function describing the mode. We will not calculate them but just show how they appear on a screen.

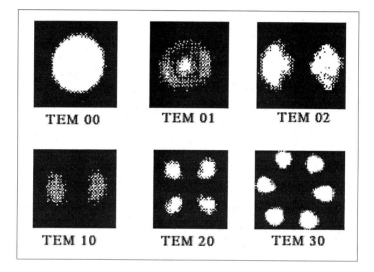

**Fig. 7:** *Transversal modes of laser radiation. Shown is the intensity distribution when one is looking into the laser. The most frequently used mode is TEMoo.*

For practical lasers the $TEM_{00}$, $TEM_{01}$ and the doughnut mode are relevant. The $TEM_{00}$ has a bell shaped Gaussian intensity distribution

$$I(x) = I_0 \cdot \exp(-(x - w)^2) \quad (17)$$

25

where $I_o$ is the intensity on the optical axis, $I(x)$ the intensity at distance x and w the width of the distribution.

## 1.2.6 Changing colors: Frequency multiplication (see also Appendix 4.4)

Most lasers provide only one or a few wavelengths. This range can be extended by the use of transparent birefringent crystals (with two optical axes). When an intense light wave impinges on such a crystal, electrons will be induced to oscillate cooperatively under the influence of the electric field in the wave. The geometry of the crystal acts as if the wave were limited by a resonator. The result is that higher harmonics occur, much like as in a string of a violin that can generate harmonic octaves of its basic tone at high excitation. In some crystals (see, for example, Box 5), for a certain wavelength range, the generation of the second harmonic can reach an efficiency of 15–20 % of the total energy of the light wave, i.e. in addition to the original laser wavelength the half wavelength will leave the crystal. The ground wave and second harmonic can be separated by a prism. In some favorable cases, the third and fourth harmonic are also generated with significant intensity. In particular, the NdYAG laser with its working wavelength of 1064 nm can thus generate additional wavelengths at 532, 355 and 266 nm. One also speaks of frequency doubled, tripled, etc. lasers. In a similar way, two beams exactly double in wavelength can be generated. The latter are used in basic quantum mechanical studies where two identical beams of light are needed; these play, however, no role in the context of this book.

**Box 5: Crystals for frequency doubling (from W. Demtröder, Laserspektroskopie, Springer 1993)**

| Chemical symbol | Common name | Wavelengths to be multiplied |
|---|---|---|
| KDP | Potassium diphosphate | 517-1500 nm |
| Urea | Urea | 473-1400 nm |
| $LiJO_3$ | Lithium iodate | 570-5500 nm |
| $\beta-BaB_2O_4$ | BBO | 400-3330 nm |
| KTP | Potassium triphosphate | 1000-2500 nm |

## 1.2.7 Real lasers

From what we have just learned about lasing a real laser is just a cylinder filled with some suitable material and a mirror at either end. Exactly! A laser is that simple! But there are still a few catches. One has to find good lasing material. The mirrors have to be exactly parallel to each other and the distance between them must match exactly the wavelength generated by the transition from the upper to the lower lasing state. In the early times of laser research it was hard work to satisfy all these conditions. But today the technology is available, and thus lasers at a price of twenty or thirty dollars can be found. The number of lasers available on the market is already so large that it would be beyond the scope of this book to mention them all. The sizes of such lasers range from microscopic to table-top lasers to factory-sized systems for nuclear fusion.

Laser media range from air to nitrogen, to other gases to semiconductors, and lasers are classed according to their medium type.

Often it is easier to build a laser with a long (red or infrared) working wavelength (though there are exceptions such as the nitrogen laser). A law in physics explains why: As we have learned, spontaneous emission competes with the stimulated emission required for the lasing process. Spontaneous emission scales with the inverse third power of the wavelength. Thus, for example, at an infrared wavelength of 10000 nm, spontaneous emission is by a factor of 8000 smaller for than green wavelengths (500 nm).

For use in industry or medicine, often the costs per Watt laser power is the critical

**Box 6: Laser classes and typical examples**

| Laser class | Typical examples |
| --- | --- |
| Solid state | Ruby, Neodym YAG, Sapphire |
| Neutral gas | Helium-Neon, Nitrogen |
| Gas ion | Argon$^+$, Krypton$^+$ |
| Metal vapor | Copper vapor |
| Semiconductor | GaInAs |
| Dye | Solutions of a large choice of dyes |
| Titanium sapphire | Tunable from 720 nm to infrared |

quantity. In such cases the $CO_2$ laser (working wavelength 10000 nm) is unbeatable: it provides kilowatt laser powers at a price of a few thousand dollars.

## Summary and outlook

With the laser as a source of intense directed light we can spatially separate the light source and the object to be analyzed or worked on. While the laser provides high intensity as compared to classical light sources, a further factor of $10^8$ can be gained by extreme focusing. The instrument for achieving such focusing is the classical light microscope.

# 1.3 Microscopes and cameras

The second ingredient for our recipe for building a laser microbeam is a classical scientific instrument: the light microscope. Light microscopy has had and still has an enormous impact on biology and medicine. It allows us to visualize fine details of living cells and to view even single molecules (see, for example sections 4 and 5 of this book). Two centuries of microscopy have made the light microscope an almost perfect optical instrument. Its typical magnification of a factor of 1000 means that, for example, a pencil, magnified to this degree, would appear as a tower 150 m in height.

## 1.3.1 Different types of light microscopy

The types of objects for microscopy can be very different. For example, objects may have different degrees of transparency. In one extreme case no light can penetrate an object at all, i.e. only its surface can be imaged. In an other extreme case the object is totally transparent, i.e. under normal conditions it cannot be seen at all. For each case, and all intermediate situations, a specific visualizing technique is available:

| | |
|---|---|
| Reflection | Non transparent objects (Material research) |
| Bright field | Amplitude objects |
| Dark field | Amplitude objects, negative display |
| Phase contrast | Transparent (Phase) objects, many objects in biology |
| Differential interference contrast | Thick phase objects |
| Fluorescence | Fluorophores |

Box 7 gives a short survey on these variants of microscopy.

### Box 7: Short survey of different types of light microscopy

#### Reflection microscopy

is in principle a surface analytical technique. Light impinges on the object, part of it is reflected and used for imaging. This type of microscopy is often used in material research, for example to inspect wafers or surfaces after laser treatment.

#### Bright field microscopy

is the standard type of microscopy in biology. Biological objects are quite often more or less transparent but have some scattering or absorbing subcellular structures. Such structures are called "amplitude objects" since they modify the intensity of the light passing through it.

#### Dark field microscopy

is also suitable for amplitude objects. Here, for illumination the secondary maxima of the Bessel function (see Appendix A3) are used for illumination. The effect is that the image appears as a type of negative of the corresponding bright field image.

#### Phase contrast microscopy

visualizes objects which are transparent but have an index of refraction (Appendix A1) different from the environment. When a light wave enters an object of higher refractive index, it is retarded by a quarter of a wavelength . This wave, after having passed the phase object, can be brought to interference (Appendix A4) with undisturbed light which is always present at suitable illumination conditions. By negative interference the phase difference is converted into an amplitude difference and the phase objects appear darker than the environment .

### Differential interference contrast (DIC)

is used for thick phase objects. In DIC, contours are made visible by an addition of different waves so that at all sites where there is a gradient in the refractive index the signal is highly amplified.

### Fluorescence microscopy

Fluorescence emission has a wavelength significantly different from the wavelength of excitation (Appendix A5). In addition, fluorescent light is emitted in all directions of space, particularly also in the direction from where the excitation light is coming. When fluorescence is observed from this side one speaks of "epifluorescence microscopy". This allows one to separate fluorescent light from the illuminating light using a filter set and on a spatial basis. Under observation conditions close to ideal, fluorescence may be observed before an almost dark background. This allows one to visualize very faint structures and even individual molecules, provided they contain a fluorophore which can be excited suitably and which re-emits fluorescence.

## 1.3.2 Object illumination

Essential in all types of microscopy is the illumination, which comes from the side opposite the direction of observation. The "Köhler illumination" (Fig. 8) is applied to illuminate the object with parallel light. For this purpose, the light source is positioned close to the focus of a lens called a "collector" since its task is to collect as much as possible of the source's light. Close to the collector is a diaphragma. This is used to regulate the total light flow to the object. A second lens, the condenser, images the light onto the object. A second diaphragma in front (on the source side) of the condensor can be used to select only those partial rays which are close to the optical axis. This costs intensity, but allows ideal illumination quality.

Other types of illumination are phase contrast illumination and fluorescence illumination. The mechanism described above for phase contrast microscopy tells only half the story. While it would work in principle, negative interference shifted by a quarter of a wavelength generates only moderate effects. Ideal negative interference occurs when the phase shift is half a wavelength. Therefore, part of the light is additionally retarded by a

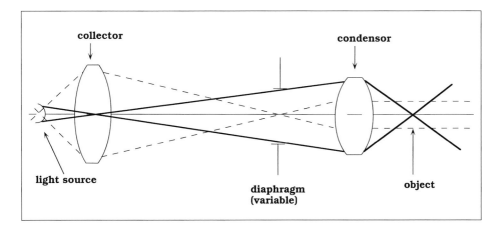

**Fig. 8:** *Köhler illumination. It fits the numerical aperture of the illumination optimally to the numerical aperture (see also Appendix A2) of the objective. The variable diaphragma is almost closed. By moving the condensor along the optical axis the diaphragma spot, observed via the objective (not shown), becomes sharp. This is the optimal Köhler illumination for the objective being used. Optimal Köhler illumination is essential for optimal resolution of the microscope, and is a prerequisite for phase contrast microscopy.*

ring-like zone in the objective which shifts the wave by another quarter of a wavelength. Only then are the two wave types brought to interference to achieve an optimal effect.

For fluorescence illumination often a mercury vapor lamp (for example HBO 50), provides a mixture of wavelengths, from which a suitable band width (5–10 nm) is chosen by optical filters. A second optical filter selecting the expected fluorescence wavelength protects additionally against unwanted stray light. Both filter types (typical designation G 365/LP 420) can be purchased in premounted housings and set into the microscope as a whole.

## 1.3.3 The magnification of a microscope

The simplest microscope is a magnifying glass. In principle it would be possible to achieve any magnification with such a single lens system. However, in order to achieve very high magnifications one would need image distances of several meters – not very practical. Therefore, microscopes consist of at least two lenses: the objective and the eyepiece. The objective produces the real image. The eyepiece, or ocular, magnifies this image further. Formally, the magnification of the microscope is

$$Magn = Magn_{objective} \cdot Magn_{eyepiece} \quad (18)$$

or, with the equations derived in appendix A2, section A2.4,

$$Magn = s_{image}/s_{object} \cdot -(1+25 \text{ cm}/f_{eyepiece}). \quad (19)$$

$s_{object}$ and $f_{eyepiece}$ should be small in order to obtain high magnifications, and $s_{image}$ is much larger. Also, $s_{object}$ is approximately $f_{objective}$ (Equation A16 in Appendix A2.4). Actually, $s_{image}$ accounts for almost the total length L of the microscope tubus. Thus one obtains an approximation formula for the overall magnification of the microscope

$$Magn = L/f_{objective}-(1+25\text{cm}/f_{eyepiece}) \quad (20)$$

which only contains quantities which can be taken from the manual of a microscope. The overall magnification has a negative sign, indicating that the overall image is upright. Since the length L of the focus is also a fixed quantity,

*the overall magnification of a real microscope is primarily determined by the focal lengths of objective and eyepiece.*

Theoretically, the magnification of a microscope can be made very large but this may not be terribly useful. A second important measure determining the quality of a microscope is how small the distance is which it can resolve between two objects. As will be shown in Appendix A2.4 this resolution is determined solely by $f_{objective}$ but not by $f_{eyepiece}$. Therefore, much effort is put into a small focal length and thus a large magnification (up to 100x) of the objective, while the magnification of the eypiece is typically 10 to 12.5x, a value which can be achieved with comparatively little effort. Thus, the limit for the overall magnification of microscopes is 1000- to 1250-fold.

## 1.3.4 A two-lens microscope

If you are not familiar with geometric constructions of optical paths but are interested in more details, refer to Appendices A1 and A2. Fig. 9 shows the imaging of a simple two-lens microscope. In real microscopes (see below) two details are dif-

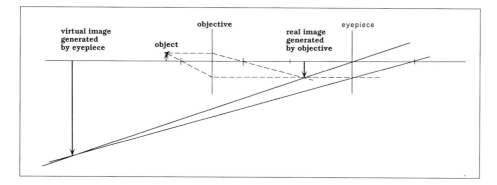

**Fig. 9:** *Imaging of a simple two lens microscope: An object, an arrow, is located at 1.5 focal lengths in front of the objective. The real image is at 3 focal lengths on the other side of the object and is double in size. This real image is closer than one focal length in front of the eyepiece. The final image is on the same side as the real image. It is therefore a virtual image which cannot be projected onto a screen but can still be observed with the eye. Its distance from the eyepiece is three times the distance of the real image from the eyepiece. Thus the final image is three times as large as the real image and six times as large as the original object.*

ferent: the object is closer to the objective's focus than in the construction of Fig. 9 and thus the magnification is larger. In addition the focal points of the objective and eyepiece are close to each other.

In the figure the objective has a focus of 2 cm, the ocular has a focus of 16 cm. The ratio of the focal lengths of the ocular and objective is 8. It is not just by accident that this is equal to the degree of magnification. We have found a general law of microscopy (see also Appendix A2).

## 1.3.5 Real microscopes

Therefore, real microscopes today are all of similar design. The focal length of the eyepiece has been chosen by experience and convention to be 160 mm. The magnification as well as the resolution are then determined mainly by the objective, which should have a focus as small as possible (except if lower than optimal resolution and magnification are required in the case of larger objects). For that reason enormous effort is put into the design of objectives and the quality of the objective determines the optical quality of the microscope. No microscope today consists of only two lenses. Fig. 10 (kindly provided by Dr.H. Gundlach, Carl Zeiss, Jena) shows two basic microscope designs.

Fig. 10 a is, in principle, the design we have used in Fig. 9. In Fig. 10 b two additional lenses can be seen: they are provided to give a stretch of parallel ray propagation. The position between the two additional lenses can be used to add other optical elements such as mirrors or filters without disturbing the imaging process. Fig. 11, finally, shows a microscope where the objective lens is replaced by a system of six lenses. This system is usually built into a separate housing and can be easily exchanged in commercial microscopes. Such a system with housing will from now on be dubbed "objective", while a simple lens will be called "objective lens".

A real microscope consists of a massive support which holds all the optical elements, the illumination elements, the imaging elements and elements to observe and record images.

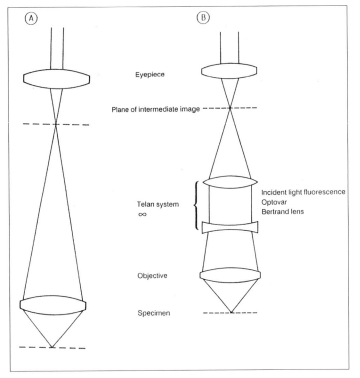

**Fig. 10:** *Schematic optical path for objectives of finite length a: Conventional microscope with finite optics b: Microscope with finite optics and two addtional lenses between which additional optical components can be inserted. (Courtesy H. Gundlach.)*

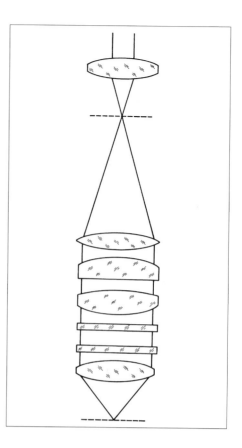

**Fig. 11:** *Schematic design of a real microscope. The objective lens is replaced by a system of lenses (bottom of the figure) which usually are mounted together in a separate housing. (Courtesy H.Gundlach.)*

## 1.3.6 Microscope objectives

Microscope objectives may consist of up to 16 lenses made of different transparent materials. They are no longer symmetrical with respect to their two overall focal lengths. Since glasses with counteracting wavelength dependencies can be used, such lens systems have highly reduced spherical and chromatic aberrations. Their quality is often the result of sophisticated numerical calculations. For more details see Appendix A1, A2. The largest magnification of microscope objectives is 100x. The high numerical apertures can be achieved only with oil (n=1.556, see Appendix A1) in the space between object and objective. Plan-apochromates have the highest numerical apertures and are available with variable apertures. Among the apochromates with highest numerical apertures of 1.4, the Nikon has the longest working distance 0.17 mm followed by Olympus 0.10 mm and Zeiss 0.08 mm.

## Box 8: Data for some selected microscope objectives

### Leica

| Magnification | Focal length on object side | Working distance object side | Image distance image side | Angular aperture object side | Numerical aperture object side |
|---|---|---|---|---|---|
| 4x | 28.3 mm | 9.5 mm | 141 mm | 11 degree | 0.10 |
| 10x | 14.8 mm | 7.1mm | 163 mm | 29 degree | 0.25 |
| 40x | 4.3 mm | 0.54 mm | 176 mm | 81 degree | 0.65 |
| 100x | 1.8 mm | 0.16 mm | 182 mm | 106 degree | 1.25 |

### Zeiss ICS

| corrected for infinite image | numerical apertures | working distances (mm) |
|---|---|---|
| 40x Plan-Neofluars | 0.75–1.30 (oil) | 0.12 (oil)–0.33 |
| 63x Neofluars (oil) | 1.25 | 0.10 |
| 100x Plan Neofluars | 1.3 | 0.06 |
| 100x Plan-Apochromates | 1.40 | 0.08 |
| 100x Achrostigmat | 1.25 | 0.25 |
| 100x Ultrafluar | 1.20 | |

### Olympus

| | | |
|---|---|---|
| 40x Universal Plan Fluorite | 0.75 | 0.51 |
| 60x Universal Plan Fluorite | 0.65–1.25 | 0.10 |
| 100x Universal Plan Fluorite | 1.30 | 0.10 |
| 100x Plan Apochromat | 1.40 | 0.10 |
| 100x Universal Planapochromat | 0.50-1.35 | 0.10 |

### Nikon

| | | |
|---|---|---|
| 40x CFI Plan Fluor | 0.75 | 0.72 |
| 60x CFI Plan Fluor | 0.85 | 0.44–0.48 |
| 100x CFI Plan Fluor | 1.30 or 0.5–1.3 | 0.20 |
| 100x CFI Plan Apochromat | 1.40 | 0.17 |

Achrostigmates have the longest working distances at a given aperture. The Leica and the Zeiss Achrostigmate have long working distances (0.16 and 0.25 mm) at numerical apertures of 1.25. Fluorescence objectives are between the former objective types. They are partially transparent for UV and are available in several magnifications for phase contrast and DIC. UV objectives are transparent for UV but have significantly poorer numerical apertures and working distances.

Unfortunately, it is impossible to produce the "ideal" objective, i.e. an objective without any disadvantages. For example, in order to construct an objective with no chromatic aberration (apochromates) one needs glasses which have a slight but for some purposes still significant intrinsic fluorescence and which have some spherical aberrations. Only recently, objectives with small chromatic and small spherical aberrations have become commercially available. (Planapochromates). In turn, for very low light level microscopy, glasses with low intrinsic fluorescence have to be used. Since the choice of different refractive indices and different wavelength dependence is not as large as for normal glasses, these objectives are not ideal with respect to aberrations. Finally, for work in the ultraviolet range, as in laser microbeam work, the objectives have to be made by quartz glass, since other glasses start to absorb light at wavelengths below 350 nm. These objectives yield a considerably poorer imaging quality.

## 1.3.7 Microscope detectors

The classical microscope detector is the human eye. It is one of the most sensitive detectors available and requires only 40 photons to generate a signal. A disadvantage is the eye's limited ability to see contrasts. In principle it reacts logarithmically to different light intensities. Photographic films, and particulary video cameras of various types, are much better suited for static detection. Also, the output signal of cameras can be recorded and re-used, and it can be digitalized for image processing.

Monochrome (black and white) as well as color cameras are used in microscopy. The light-sensitive part is arranged as a matrix of picture elements (pixels). The standard arrangement, as in consumer cameras for home use is approx. 500x700 pixels. However, a large number of other standards exist in cameras for scientific use and it is a science in itself to select the optimal camera for a given type of experiment. The following is a checklist for such a selection procedure. Certainly it is subjective, but it may serve at least as a first guide:

Checklist for camera selection

*Is a color camera really required?*
The cheapest monochrome camera is often better than comparatively expensive color cameras. Often it is better to image a colored object by using a monochrome camera, different optical filters and pseudo colors to generate a two-or three-color picture.

*In what wavelength range does the signal come?*
CCD cameras are fashionable and reasonably priced, but they work better on the red side of the visible spectrum than in the blue. For the latter it is better to take a more expensive tube camera (for example Chalnikon), which in turn decreases in sensitivity for red wavelengths.

*Are the objects static for approximately 10 seconds?*
With static objects one can use slow scan cameras which collect and thereby integrate signal over some time. Such cameras are very sensitive at a reasonable price.

*The remaining choices:*
For fast, low light objects there remains the single photon camera, which is basically a matrix of amplified micro-photomultipliens. Its spatial resolution is often poorer than that of consumer cameras and it is available only as a monochrome camera.

## Summary and outlook

The light microscope allows us to conveniently observe living objects. It is a standard technique of biology and medicine and thus it is one ideal component of the laser microtools we want to develop. Optical properties such as the resolution of the microscope are mainly determined by the numerical aperture of the objective, a combination of up to 16 lenses.

## Selected literature

H. Gundlach (1994) Microscopy, in: Ullmanns Encyclopedia of Industrial Chemistry, VCH Weinheim

## 1.4 Laser microbeams and optical tweezers

Now you have all the parts together to build laser microbeams and or optical tweezers. You just have to combine a microscope with suitable lasers. Then you will have a tool in your hands which will allow you, with table-top equipment, to perform tasks otherwise possible only with factory-sized machines or to perform experiments which are not possible with any other tool at all. Examples are:

- generating heat at levels matching those existing on the sun,
- causing objects to accelerate without any mechanical contact,
- working in the interior of closed objects,
- manipulating microscopic objects, and measuring forces with pico-newton accuracy.

The laser micrcobeam is a tool for pricking, cutting or welding biological and biomedical objects. This requires a strong absorption of the laser light by biological material. Microbeams are occasionally also called optical scissors (Liang et al., 1994). For recent reviews see Kasuya and Tsukakoshi, 1989, Berns et al., 1991, Greulich and Weber, 1992, Weber and Greulich, 1992, Hoyer et al., 1996.

In contrast, optical tweezers are used for gentle handling of biological objects. This requires a different wavelength range, and moderate laser powers. A number of different terms are used in the literature to describe almost the same device, lasers using light pressure and gradient forces for manipulation of microscopic objects:

- optical trap,
- (single beam gradient) laser trap,
- optical tweezers,
- photonic tweezers, and
- laser tweezers.

Sometimes even the expression "microbeam" is used, but this may be confused with the pulsed microbeam used for micromachining and thus should be avoided. The expressions "single beam gradient laser trap" and "optical tweezers" are synonymous. The expressions "optical tweezers" and "optical trap" are those of the inventor of this technique, A. Ashkin, and will be used in this book. Reviews are available from Wright et al. (1990), Chu (1991), Svoboda and Block (1994), Ashkin

(1997) and the three reviews mentioned in the context of laser microbeams. If you are interested in quick information, see the short reviews of Pool (1990), Block (1992), Kuo and Sheetz (1992), Greulich (1992), Simmons and Finer (1993), Schütze and Clement-Sengewald (1994), Monajembashi et al. 1997. Two videofilms show laser micromanipulation experiments in motion (Greulich et al., 1995, Schütze et al. 1996). A book on optical tweezers appeared in 1998 (Sheetz, 1998).

## 1.4.1 Choice of the laser

For microbeams, pulsed ultraviolet lasers are particularly suitable (see Section 2.2). In contrast, optical tweezers should be used only to exert forces requiring light pressure (Section 1.1.5); and thus require other lasers. This is discussed in more detail in Sections 2.4 and 2.5. For optical tweezers, absorption of light by biological objects should be as small as possible. Continuous infrared lasers of moderate power are optimally suited for that purpose.

Such a choice was not possible in early times of laser microbeam research. Visible lasers such as the red pulsed ruby laser or the green continuous argon ion laser had to be used. Today, an affordable ultraviolet laser is the nitrogen laser with a working wavelength of 337 nm and a typical pulse duration from 0.5 up to 5 ns. Pulse energies are of the order of several hundred microjoules (for the definition of energy units see Box 2), the pulse repetition rates are between 1 and 20 pulses per second. Other lasers for microbeams are excimer lasers or excimer-pumped dye lasers as well as frequency doubled or tripled NdYAG (Neodymium Yttrium Aluminium Garnet) lasers. Probably the most versatile, though expensive, microbeam laser is the Titanium Sapphire laser with subpicosecond pulses and variable wavelength.

For optical tweezers, NdYAG lasers (1064 nm), NdYLF lasers (1047/1953 nm) InGaAsP semiconductor lasers (1330 nm) and continuous wave Titanium Sapphire lasers have been primarily used so far. With respect to the choice of lasers for optical tweezers one problem should be realized: the interaction of these lasers is highly dependent on the specific wavelength. Thus, specific experience with each new laser type will have to be accumulated with regard to possible laser damage (see Section 2.3). Best known are the effects of the NdYAG laser at 1064 nm. (For the laser types see also Box 9.)

**Box 9: Typical parameters of lasers used in microbeams and optical tweezers**

| Lasing medium | Wave-length | Average power | Pulse width | Pulse energy | Pulses/sec | Remark |
|---|---|---|---|---|---|---|
| Excimer | 308 nm | 10 W | 20 ns | 100 mJ | 200 | primary UV source |
| Nitrogen | 337 nm | 1 W | 5 ns | 200 µJ | 20 | should be diffraction-limited. |
| Argon | 514 nm | 10 W | continuous | – | | |
| Ruby | 694 nm | small | 30 ns | | <<1 | first laser used |
| NdYLF | 1047 nm | | continuous | | | |
| NdYAG | 1064 nm | 10 W | 5 ns | 100 mJ | 30 | doubled, tripled etc. |
| NdYAG | 1064 nm | 1 W | in traps: continuous | – | | diode pumped version easy to operate |
| InGaAs | 780 nm | 0.1 W | in traps: continuous | | | compact laser |
| MOPA | 985 nm | 1 W | | | | |
| InGaAsP | 1330 nm | 0.1 W | in traps: continuous | – | | compact laser |
| TiSapphire | variable | | 100 fs | | | tunable, extremely short pulse |

## 1.4.2 Choice of microscope and objective

A fluorescence microscope is recommendable, i.e. a microscope with two illumination paths. Almost any fluorescence microscope can be used to build a laser microbeam or optical tweezers. With standard (upright) fluorescence microscopes there are some restrictions in handling the specimens. Therefore, if you have free choice, use an inverted microscope. But if you have only an upright version, don't hesitate to use it. A large variety of experiments can be performed with this type of microscope. The only restriction is that the mirror close to the objective should move with the objective during focusing, since the distance between it and the image side of the objective should remain constant. Some microscopes do not satisfy this requirement and should therefore be avoided.

The following microscopes have been used or suggested for use in laser microbeams and/or optical tweezers, but this list does not mean that other microscopes are not suitable.

- Olympus IMT 2 with Plan 100 x, NA=1.2
- Zeiss IM 35, Axiovert 135 with Neofluar 100 x, NA=1.3
- Leica DMIRB: PL Fluotar 100x, NA=1.3
- Nikon Diaphot 300

Since in microbeams, albeit not in optical tweezers, wavelengths and pulse intensities are chosen for strong interaction with matter, you will also have unwanted

**Box 10: Pros and cons for using quartz or glass objectives in microbeams**

|  | Quartz objective and small laser | Normal objective and larger laser |
| --- | --- | --- |
| Loss of light | small | high |
| Damage to objective | small | high |
| Costs for objective | high | smaller |
| Cost for laser media and maintenance | low | high |
| Types of microscopy possible | restricted*) (for example DIC not possible) | no significant limitation |

*) The choice of possible microscopy types may not be as restrictive as it appears: By using a UV objective for microirradiation and any other type of objective in the objective revolver of the microscope, one may switch between the two, provided one can work dry, i.e. without immersion fluid. Only when such a fluid prevents fast switching or when the time between irradiation and observation has to be shorter than a few seconds, this switching is not possible and switching between different types of microscopy becomes difficult.

interactions with the optical elements, particularly with the objective. Thus the objective should be transparent for UV. Glass optics will be sufficiently transparent for the nitrogen laser in order not to damage seriously the objective. But there will be losses in intensity. On the other hand, quartz optics is transparent, but a 100 x quartz objective will cost several thousands of dollars.

Thus you have to optimize your decision. Box 10 lists some advantages and disadvantages of using UV or glass objective.

## 1.4.3 Building a microbeam and/or optical tweezers

Before you start building a laser microbeam or optical tweezers, you have to make a basic decision. Do you want to build it with a fixed beam. Then you need an x-y stage (ideally a motor-driven xy object stage with at least 0.125 micrometer resolution) for your microscope. Relative motion is generated by moving the object with this stage. Alternatively, you may use a movable (flying) beam. Then you need adjustable mirrors in the path of the laserbeam between laser and objective. Which approach is the best depends on the experiments to be performed. The fixed beam version is more advisable for microbeams alone and often for microbeams combined with optical tweezers. In fact the majority of applications described in this book have been performed with fixed beams. For optical tweezers, particularly when sophisticated force measurements are planned, the flying beam version has some advantages.

Nevertheless, the construction of a laser microbeam or of optical tweezers is conceptually simple. The heart of the apparatus is a fluorescence microscope, i.e. a microscope with illumination from the direction of observation (epifluorescence illumination). In summary, you should proceed as follows:

- use an (inverted) fluorescence microscope,
- replace standard optics with UV optics (for microbeam only),
- add two semitransparent mirrors in the fluorescence illumination path, and
- couple, via the mirrors, a pulsed UV laser and a
- continuous IR laser, with the fluorescence illumination
- path and focus them via the objective.

## 1.4.4 The coupling unit

Two approaches are possible to couple the laser(s) into the optical path. One uses the path for bright field illumination. In this case an additional (expensive) high numerical aperture objective (NA>1, 63x or 100x) will be required. The other approach simply couples the laser to the fluorescence path. A three-path mirror or a semipermeable mirror inserted into the optical path allows simultaneous microbeam work and fluorescence observation. For optical tweezers you may couple the laser(s) directly by mirrors or via an optical fiber (occasionally in the literature fibers are said to be unsuitable, but this may be a matter of preference). The high power laser of a microbeam should be coupled directly. Fig. 12 (modified from Monajembashi and Greulich 1995) depicts the details.

Since the aim is to focus such a laser up to the highest theoretically possible limit, i.e. to the diffraction limit, the aperture on the side of the image of the microscope objective (which is often called the "exit pupil") has to be fully illuminated by the laser. The laser beam (2 mm x 2 mm for a nitrogen laser) is expanded by a pair of lenses resembling a simple telecope, in order to exactly illuminate the lower aperture of the microscope objective.

The lens with $f_2$=150 mm is already part of many microscopes. The distance and the focal length of the second lens, added externally into the path of the laser, can be calculated as

$$D = d\, f_2/f_1. \quad (21)$$

By moving the external lens in the direction of the optical axis, the focused beam can be located above, in or below the object plane of the microscope. Correspondingly, moving this lens perpendicularly, the focused beam can be moved in the object plane. The beam expansion has an additional advantage: until the laser enters the microscope objective, its power density is moderate, i.e. the possibility of damage to optical elements is partially eliminated.

The expanded laser beam is focused by the objective. When the aperture on the image side of the objective is illuminated properly, the beam will be diffraction-limited.

At the side of the object facing the objective, the focused intensity is already sufficient enough to damage it. When a microscope objective, after prolonged use in a microbeam, is itself inspected in a stereo microscope of moderate magnification, traces of damage can be seen. These, however, do not significantly diminish the imaging properties of the objective.

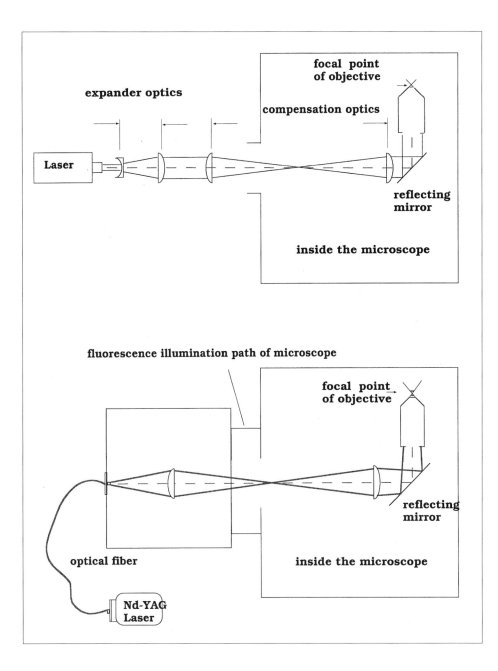

**Fig. 12:** *Upper part. Details of the coupling unit: the expander optics prepares the beam for optimal focusing and is required in any type of laser microtool. The compensation optics is only required in microscopes which already have a lens built in the illumination path. Lower part. Coupling via a glass fiber (for optical tweezers only).*

In some microscope types there is a certain area close to the objective where additional optical elements can be inserted by the user. Here attenuators (neutral density filter wedges for variation of the laser power, polarizers and shutters can be inserted, in case they cannot be immediately mounted in front of the laser outside the microscope.

High power coating of the optical elements for optimal reflection (see Appendix A1) is advisable since standard low power coatings are usually degraded after a few thousand laser pulses. (This is not necessary for tweezers.)

### 1.4.5 Mounting the parts and adjusting the lasers

Once you have all the parts together, how do you have to combine them?

For each application and for each type of microscope there is a slightly different approach required, but some general rules hold. It is useful to have a metal ground plate approximately 0.5 m x 1m. Connect your microscope firmly to the front end of the plate. Remove the fluorescence filter sets, and replace the mirror with a suitably coated one. Insert the additional lenses as described in the previous section. Mount your laser(s) on the rear part. Usually, two or three mirrors on x-y moveable holders are required to bring the laser beams into the rear entrance, where usually the fluorescence illumination lamp is located. Cover the entrance with a piece of paper and start your UV laser. The paper will act as a screen and wavelength converter which, due to a blueish fluorescence, will make the ultraviolet beam visible. For the infrared laser you need a special paper which you may purchase from many optics companies.

Adjust the laser (s) to the center of the rear entrance. Remove the paper sheets. Look to see what is coming out of the objective. You will see nothing! It is clear that your adjustment is still too coarse. Remove the objective and put your sheet of paper on the microscope stage. Then you will probably find the beam. Adjust it by changing the positions of the mirrors between the laser(s) and microscope to the center. Insert an objective of small magnification and repeat the adjustment. Finally insert the high magnification objective and do the fine adjustment. Now you have the beam in the center of the xy stage, but not yet in the correct z position. This can be adjusted by shifting the free lens of the expander telescope along the z axis (along the direction of beam propagation).

## 1.4.6 "Flying spot" – and multiple beam optical tweezers

Building optical tweezers is easier than building microbeams since at the wavelengths of tweezers optical elements are highly transparent. Thus, certain precautions against high power damage to optical elements are not necessary with optical tweezers. This means that the "flying spot" version can be more easily realized than with a microbeam. There are four ways to realize a moveable spot. In each case, one optical element in the path of the laser is moved and thus changes the direction of the beam. Often, elements of galvanometers are useful. The steering can be performed by a computer and thus complex figures can be circumscribed by the spot. Fig. 13, reproduced from Svoboda and Block, 1994, summarizes the four possibilities.

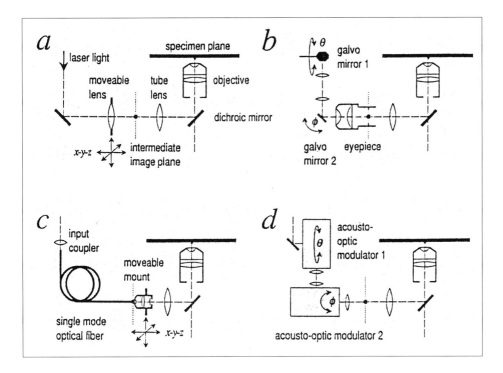

**Fig. 13:** *Four ways to scan the position of the laser spot in an optical trap in the object plane. a: Translating the moveable lens. b: Rotating galvanometer mirrors. c: Translating the end of an optical fiber. d: Deflecting the beam with an acousto optic modulator (AOM). (From: Svoboda and Block, 1994.)*

Often, elongated microscopic objects such as filamentous structures have to be held or fixed at two distant positions. In studies on cell membranes even three contact points are required (see, for example, the studies on red blood cell membranes reported in Section 6.4.2) For these purposes, double or multiple beam tweezers (Visscher and Brakenhoff, 1993) have been developed. Such double or multibeam tweezers are created essentially by adding an additional switchable mirror into "flying spot" tweezers which switches the beam from one position to the other. The two (or more) beams undergo a sort of time-sharing of the single laser available as light source.

### 1.4.7 Combination of laser microbeam and optical tweezers

For complete micromanipulation by light a combination of a microbeam with optical tweezers is required: the objects can then be held or transported with the tweezers and they can be micromanipulated with the microbeam. Such combinations have been used or reviewed, for example, by Greulich et al., 1989, Berns et al., 1991, Misawa et al., 1991 and Weber and Greulich, 1992. Fig. 14 shows one of these combinations.
In order to give you an idea of the size of the lasers, Fig. 15 shows the two lasers in comparison with a well-known size standard.

### Summary and outlook

You have now some basic information on how to build laser microtools and you have received a glimpse at the underlying physical principles. Light is a carrier of energy and of momentum and these two properties are exploited in laser microtools, which can be built by adding a pulsed ultraviolet and/or a continuous infrared laser to a fluorescence microscope. This basic knowledge allows you to perform and interpret simple experiments with laser microbeams and optical tweezers. For example, if you want to use a laser microbeam just for microperforation of cell walls or for the induction of cell fusion, it is not mandatory to know all quantitative details of interactions with biological tissue. Similarly, you can use optical tweezers as a sort of black box when you want to move or store cells or subcellular structures.

In order to exploit the full potential of laser microtools, however, you need a more quantitative knowledge of the interactions of light with living matter. In a

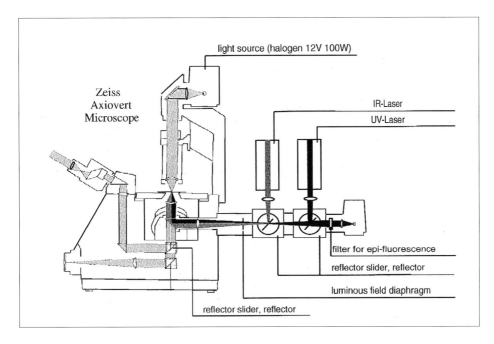

**Fig.14:** *Schematic representation of a combination of a laser microbeam with optical tweezers. In this system the fluorescence illumination lamp is still present and the two lasers are added via a semi-transparent mirror.*

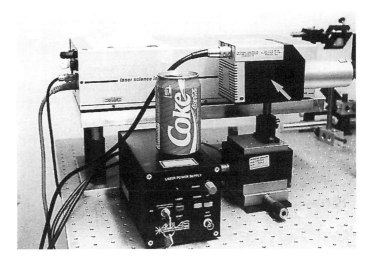

**Fig. 15:** *A nitrogen laser used for the laser microbeam (rear part) and a NdYAG laser for the optical trap (white arrow) mounted on the ground plate of the microtool apparatus. On the right (not shown) the microscope is mounted.*

number of experiments, it is not sufficient to know simply how the technique works. You need to know how much effect is generated quantitatively. For example, when using a laser microbeam, you probably want to know not only that the spot is very hot. You may wish to know *how* hot it is and what harm it is doing to your biological sample. With the optical tweezers you may not only be interested in the fact that light can exert forces. You may also want to know how strong these forces are – how they can be used quantitatively in the world of biology and medicine.

If you want this information now, you should read Sections 2.1 through 2.6. In case you would prefer to use laser microbeams and optical tweezers just as black boxes, you may, for the time being, immediately proceed to Section 3.1 and come back to Section 2.1 through 2.6 at a later time.

## Selected literature

A. Ashkin (1997) Optical trapping and manipulation of neutral particles using lasers. Proc. Natl. Acad. Sci. 94, 4853–4860.

M.W. Berns, W.H. Wright and R. Wiegand Steubing (1991) Laser microbeam as a tool in cell biology. Int. Rev. Cytol 129, 1–44.

S.M. Block (1992) Making light work with optical tweezers. Nature 360, 493-495.

S. Chu (1991) Laser manipulation of atoms and particles. Science 253, 861–866.

K.O. Greulich (1992) Moving particles by light: No longer science fiction. Royal Microscopy Society Proceedings 27, 3–10.

K.O. Greulich, G. Weber (1992) The light microscope on its way from an analytical to a preparative tool. J. Microscopy 167(2), 127–151.

K.O Greulich, U. Bauder, S. Monajembashi, N. Ponelies, S. Seeger and J. Wolfrum (1989) UV Laser Mikrostrahl und optische Pinzette (UV laser microbeam and optical tweezers). Labor 2000, 36–42.

K.O. Greulich, A. Harim, G. Leitz, N. Endlich, M. Schliwa, O. Müller, E. Schnepf, G. Weber, K. Schütze, H. Gundlach and G. Kerlen (1995), Videofilm: Laser microbeam and optical tweezers: Physical principles and application in cell biology and biotechnology. Institute for the Scientific Film, Göttingen, Germany.

C. Hoyer, S. Monajembashi and K.O. Greulich (1996) Light as a microtool: Laser microbeams and optical tweezers. Science Progress, 93.6, 233–254.

H. Misawa, M. Koshoka, K. Sasaki, N. Kitamura and H. Masuhara (1991) Three dimensional optical trapping and laser ablation of a single polymer latex particle. J. Appl. Phys. 70, 3829–3836.

S. Monajembashi, C. Hoyer and K.O. Greulich (1997) Laser microbeams and optical tweezers convert the microscope into a versatile microtool. Microscopy and Analysis, 97.1, 7–9.

T. Kasuya, and M. Tsukakoshi (1989) Laser microirradiation of cells, V.S. Letokhov, C.V. Shank and H. Walther Harwood (eds.), London. In: Laser Science and Technology Vol 1: pp 1–80.

S.C. Kuo and M.P. Sheetz (1992) Optical tweezers in cell biology. Trends in Cell Biol. 2, 116-118.

H. Liang, W.H. Wright, C.L. Rieder, E.D. Salmon, G. Profeta, J. Andrews, Y. Liu, G.J. Sonek and M.W. Berns (1994) Directed movement of chromosome arms and fragments in mitotic newt lung cells using optical scissors and optical tweezers. Exptl. Cell Res. 213, 308–312.

S. Monajembashi and K.O. Greulich (1995) Laser microbeams and optical tweezers: How they work and why they work. Progress in Biomedical Optics, SPIE paper 2628-20.

R. Pool (1990) Making Light Work of Cell Surgery. Science 248, 29–31.

K. Schütze, A. Clement-Sengewald (1994) Catch and Move – Cut or Fuse. Nature 368, 667–669.

K. Schütze, A. Clement-Sengewald, F.D. Berg, G. Brehm, R. Schütze (1995) Institute for the Scientific Film, Göttingen, Germany Videofilm: Laser microbeam and optical tweezers: Micromanipulation of gametes and embryos

M.P. Sheets ed. (1998) Laser tweezers in cell biology. In: Methods in cell biology, Academic Press.

R.M. Simmons, J.T. Finer (1993) Curr. Biol. 3, 309–311, Glasperlenspiel II: Optical tweezers.

K. Svoboda, S.M. Block (1994) Ann.Rev.Biophys. Biomol.Struct., 247–285, Biological applications of optical forces.

K. Visscher, G.J. Brakenhoff, J.J. Krol (1993) Cytometry 14, 105–114, Micromanipulation by multiple optical traps created by a single fast scanning trap integrated with the bilateral confocal scanning microscope.

G. Weber, K.O. Greulich (1992) Int. Review of Cytology 133, 1–41 Manipulation of cells, organelles and genomes by laser microbeam and optical trap.

W.H. Wright, G.J. Sonek, Y. Tadir, M.W. Berns (1990) IEEE J. Quant. Electronics 26, 2148–2157, Laser trapping in cell biology.

# Why and how light can be used as a microtool

Lasers can be hot. Perhaps you experienced this yourself. In industrial processes as well as in medical surgery this fact is exploited routinely. But what temperatures are generated exactly? Hundreds of degrees? Thousands of degrees? Perhaps even ten thousand degrees? The surprise is: it can be even much more than that. Even with comparatively small-table top lasers, extreme temperatures and a new physical state of matter, plasma can be generated.

## 2.1 Pulsed laser microbeams

### 2.1.1 Pulsed lasers can be focused to extreme intensities

There are dramatic differences between continuous and pulsed laser light. In this section only pulsed lasers will be discussed. In section 2.2 the interaction of such pulsed lasers with matter is addressed. Subsequently, section 2.3 will show you corresponding effects of continuous lasers. It will facilitate the reading of the following pages, if you remember the difference between energy, power and intensity. If you are not sure about these quantities, refer to Box 2.

Extreme intensities can be obtained by focusing a pulsed laser. Lasers used in microbeams typically generate nanosecond pulses. Each single pulse provides an energy of micro- to millijoules only. But it provides this energy in pulses of nanosecond duration. When such a laser generates, say, 1000 pulses per second, it will, within one second, deliver millijoule up to joules in energy, i.e. its average power is milliwatt up to one watt. This is not very much as compared to, for example, 40 to 100 watts produced by a standard light bulb. The situation is totally different when we ask what is the maximum power at a given instant during a pulse. Remember that the pulse duration is only nanoseconds. And a millijoule per nanosecond is a peak power of a megawatt!

But that is not yet all. We are not really interested in the power but in the power per area (=intensity). Since we can focus laser light into a spot of submicrometer dimensions, while laser beams have cross sections of square millimetres, we can concentrate laser light by a factor of $10^6$ to $10^8$. A detailed calculation is given in Box 11.

### Box 11: Power concentration by focusing in a microscope

When a laser is absorbed by material, heat is generated. By focusing light, enormous power densities can be generated, particularly when pulsed lasers are used. In Appendix A3 you will learn that, using a microscope objective with an aperture of 1.4, a laser can be focused to a diameter of approx. 7/8 $\lambda$. This is the diameter of the "Airy disc" (see Appendix A3). Strictly, only 84% of the power is concentrated there. For the estimate below this value will be set at 100%.

For a nitrogen laser ($\lambda$=337 nm) this is approx. 295 nm and corresponds to a cross sectional area of approx. 1/15 $\mu m^2$. The reciprocal of this is $15 \cdot 10^8$ cm$^{-2}$ and is a measure for the increase in power density by focusing.

A nitrogen laser providing pulses of 1 microjoule at a pulse duration of 0.5 ns has a peak power of approx.

$$10^{-6} \text{ J} / 0.5 \cdot 10^{-9} \text{ sec} = 2 \cdot 10^3 \text{ W} = 2 \cdot 10^3 \text{ W} = 2 \text{ kW}.$$

The power density (intensity) is then

$$I = 2 \cdot 10^3 \text{ W} \cdot 15 \cdot 10^8 / \text{cm}^2 = 3 \cdot 10^{12} \text{ W/cm}^2.$$

Thus, an extremely high intensity can be obtained with a comparably small and affordable laser such as a nitrogen laser.

For a continuous NdYAG laser (wavelength 1064 nm) the smallest diameter is 930 nm, the cross section area 0.68 $\mu m^2$, the focusing factor $1.5 \cdot 10^8$. With 0.1 Watt the intensity is

$$I = 0.1 \text{ W} \cdot 1.5 \cdot 10^8 / \text{cm}^2$$

$$I = 1.5 \cdot 10^7 \text{ W/cm}^2.$$

**Box 12: Powers and power densities with classical light sources and with lasers**

| Power | 1 Watt | |
|---|---|---|
| | = 1 Joule per second | |
| | | |
| Laserpointer | 0.5 | Milliwatt |
| Light bulb | 15 to 200 | Watt |
| Heating power of a man | 50 | Watt |
| $CO_2$ Laser (continuous) | 5 | Kilowatt |
| Automobile | 50-100 | Kilowatt |
| Wind driven power station | 1 | Megawatt |
| Nuclear power station | 1 | Gigawatt |
| Short pulsed laser, peak | 1 | Terawatt |
| but: average power of this laser | a few | Milliwatt |

| Intensity | Watt per cm² | |
|---|---|---|
| | | |
| 60 Watt bulb at a distance of 1 m | 0.00001 | ($10^{-5}$) |
| Sunshine at Earths surface | 0.1 | ($10^{-1}$) |
| Continuous focused laser | 1 Bio | ($10^{9}$) |
| Pulsed focused laser | 1 Trio | ($10^{21}$) |

## 2.1.2 Bringing the Sun into the lab

Box 12 gave us some values for intensities which can be generated in laser microbeams. You may be impressed by the sheer numbers themselves. You will perhaps be even more impressed when you see what temperatures are generated by such intensities. A surprisingly simple sequence of arguments will give us an idea of these dramatic effects. The temperature generated by a laser is related to the intensity (i.e. to the power per area). In the following discussion we will assume that a laser pulse is fully absorbed in a layer of a wavelength thickness. We will later have to go a little bit more into details. For sufficiently short pulse durations (nanoseconds or less) one can assume that

1   the energy is deposited in the material (within nanoseconds);
2   during energy deposition (i.e. within nanoseconds) no heat flow occurs, i.e. for the time of absorption, the material is thermally isolated; and
3   after energy deposition the heat expands in a shock wave with at least the speed of sound (in aqueous solution: 1 km/s or 1 mm/ns).

Assumption 1 is trivial – energy can be deposited only as long as the laser pulse lasts. Assumption 2 is, at least, reasonable. Thermal relaxation times at temperature differences below 100 degrees last microseconds. This time is much longer than the laser pulse and there is not enough time for heat flow during the laser pulse. Assumption 3 can be made in a type of iterative reasoning: solely with assumptions 1 and 2 will it be shown that the temperature rise is drastic. The speed of heat flow is dependent on the temperature difference, which will, at sufficiently high values, reach a saturation value – the speed of sound in the given medium.

A very naive approach can make plausible that even a laser pulse of 1 µJoule and 0.5 ns duration will cause a dramatic temperature rise. It is assumed that the pulse is fully absorbed in the focus which has a diameter of 295 nm (this is the diameter which can be obtained by focusing a typical microbeam laser, see appendix A3. Its depth is also assumed to be 295 nm. The volume of the focus is then approximately 1/50 fl. If the absorber is water ($1/50$ fl $= 1/50 \cdot 10^{-12}$ g) the estimate (Box 8) gives an extremely high value for the temperature.

### Box 13: Estimation of the temperature generated by a laser pulse

1 calorie (4.13 J) heats 1 ml water by 1 °C (definition of the calorie)

1 µcalorie (4.13 µJ) heats 1 ml water by $10^{-6}$ °C (a millionth of a degree)

1 µcalorie (4.13 µJ) heats $(1/50) \cdot 10^{-12}$ g water by $50 \cdot 10^6$ °C

The result that a few µJ are sufficient to heat water by tens of millions of degrees Centigrade is so incredible that we have to question where we have made an error. Correct is that a microjoule, absorbed totally in a microscope focus would indeed provide an incredible amount of energy per volume. However, from Box 19 in Section 2.3.1 it will be seen that the penetration depth of the nitrogen laser wavelength in biological tissue is 60 µm. Using the Lambert Beer law (see appendix, Section A5.5) one can calculate that in a layer of 295 nm depth only 0.5% of the incoming energy is deposited. The consequence is that we have to repeat the estimate above with this fraction of energy. The result is a temperature rise of 250000 °C – still surprisingly high. In box 14 a more professional estimate is made using the «Stefan Boltzmann law» for black body radiation. It will give a surprisingly high temperature, too.

## Box 14: Heat and power density : Use of the Stefan Boltzmann law.

The Stefan Boltzmann law allows one to calculate the power density which is emitted by a thermal source. When the power density is known, the temperature can be calculated. For example, the sun's radiation density on the Earth's surface can be measured. It is 1345 W/m$^2$. The Sun's surface is 0.696 million km from the center of the Sun, the Earth's orbit around the Sun at 149.6 million km, i.e. at 214 Sun radii. Thus the power density at the Sun's surface is $214^2 = 45796$ times higher, i.e.

$$I = 45796 \cdot 1345 \text{ W/m}^2 = 6.16 \cdot 10^7 \text{ W/m}^2.$$

Using the Stefan Boltzmann law

$$I = \sigma \cdot T^4$$

with s=$5.67 \cdot 10^{-8}$ W/(m$^2$K$^4$) the temperature at the Sun's surface can be calculated as

$$T = {}_4\sqrt{I/s} = {}_4\sqrt{(6.16 \cdot 10^7/5.67 \cdot 10^{-8})}$$

$$T = {}_4\sqrt{1090 \cdot 10^{12}} = 5.74 \cdot 10^3 \text{ °K} = 5746 \text{ °C.}$$

Correspondingly, the heat generated by complete absorption of a given laser power density can be calculated. For example, a laser pulse of 1 ns duration with an energy of 1 µJ focused to 1 micrometer ($10^{-8}$ cm$^2$) corresponds to $10^{11}$ W/cm$^2$ or $10^{17}$ W/m$^2$: Thus

$$T = {}_4\sqrt{(10^{17}/5.67 \cdot 10^{-8})} = {}_4\sqrt{18 \cdot 10^{24}} \approx 2 \text{ mio °K.}$$

Certainly this is only an upper limit, since even in strong absorbers only a part of the power is absorbed exactly at the surface and heat flow starts immediately. Also, such high temperatures have to be carefully defined. But even an error by a factor of 10000 concerning energy actually absorbed due to only partial absorption by transparent biological material will result only in a factor of 10 in temperature. In transparent biological material the true value will be considerably smaller. Nevertheless, the estimate shows that the naive estimate in the main text gives a reasonable impression of the laser – tissue interaction.

## 2.1.3 Why is the laser microbeam so precise: The heat is absorbed immediately

Even in the case that our estimates are incorrect by one or two orders of magnitude, it remains clear that very high temperatures are generated. This is hard to reconcile with the idea that the laser beam is a gentle tool. The heat effect, however, is very local. In Box 15 it is shown that the energy density of the hot spot is reduced to 1/1000 of its intial value within a few nanoseconds. In Section 2.2 you will see that this is fast enough to leave biological material which is not directly hit by the laser pulse almost undamaged.

The real uncertainty in all the estimates above is the speed of heat absorption. Certainly in the first nanoseconds after the laser pulse, heat absorption proceeds with the speed of sound. However, when due to this process, the temperature has decreased to a few hundred degrees centigrade, the speed of the final process will decline and finally the normal laws of thermal conduction become valid. There, thermal relaxation times of microseconds have been measured. However, several experiments described in the second part of this book will indeed show that the thermal damage is low and viability of cells and chromosomes is hardly affected by treatment with a few laser pulses.

## 2.1.4 The electric fields are also impressive

Light is not only a carrier of energy but also of electric field. As is the temperature, the electric field carried by light is related to the intensity I by equation 22:

$$E^2 = 2 \cdot I/(\varepsilon_o \cdot c); \quad (22)$$

where $\varepsilon_o = 8.85 \cdot 10^{-14}$ Asec/Vcm is the permittivity constant of the vacuum.

An intensity of 1 W/cm$^2$ corresponds to an electric field of 28 V/cm. Such a field can be produced when a car battery is connected to two conducting metal plates isolated from each other and separated by 0.5 cm. In turn, a focused laser with 1014 W/cm2 generates an electric field of

$$28 \cdot 10^7 \text{ V / cm} \quad (23)$$

and this corresponds to the electric field in the electron cloud of many molecules.

**Box 15: Decrease of microbeam energy density in water with the speed of sound**

*Assumption: An energy E is deposited in a spherical droplet of water (or aqueous solution) with radius r, i. e. into a volume $V=4/3\pi\, r^3=4.19\, r^3$*

When this droplet is heated to a very high temperature by putting an energy E into the volume V, the energy density is

$$D = E/4.19\ r^3.$$

Since a very sharp temperature gradient prevails , the hot spot will expand rapidly with at least the speed of sound, v. The spot radius r(t) at a given time t will be

$$r(t) = r+v\cdot t.$$

The energy per volume, D is also a function of time

$$D(t) = E/4.19\ (r+v\cdot t)^3.$$

When we define

$$F(t) = D/D(t)$$

$$F(t) = (r+v\cdot t)^3/r^3$$

$$F(t) = 1+(v\cdot t/r)^3$$

we can, by simple rearrangement of the last equation, calculate the time it takes for the energy density to be reduced to a given fraction F(t)

$$t = (r/v\ )\cdot_3\sqrt{(F(t)\text{-}1)}.$$

For example, the time at which the energy density is diluted by a factor of 1000000 is then approx.

$$t_{1000000} = 10\cdot r/v.$$

In water where the velocity of sound is 1 km/s or 1 µm/ns, one can set (r/v) in mm and obtain the time t in ns. When r at the beginning of the experiment is 0.3 mm (focusing by a microscope)

$$t_{1000000} = 30 \text{ ns.}$$

When it is 10 µm (focusing by a lens) is diluted by a factor of 1 000 000 after

$$t_{1000000} = 1 \text{ µs.}$$

## 2.1.5 Caution: X-rays

Perhaps you were surprised to learn that temperatures of up to millions of degrees centigrade are found in the center of the spot of a laser microbeam. But that is not yet all. The microbeam also generates X rays: when the atoms and molecules in plasma recombine and when electrons return to their ground state, radiation is emitted. Part of this radiation can be seen as a white to blue flash. However, when the high speed electrons in the plasma are decelerated to small velocity, they also emit «Bremsstrahlung». This effect is already significant at $10^{12}$ Watt/cm$^2$, a power density which is easily generated by laser microbeams. When such a power density impinges on a silicon surface, up to 20% of the energy is converted into X-rays with an energy of 300 electron volt (as if it had passed an electric tension of 300 volts). This corresponds to a wavelength of some ten nanometers (X-rays used in medical imaging correspond to ten thousand or more electron volts). Probably, a short soft X-ray flash does not seriously affect your biological sample. But when you have strange effects in your experiment, don't forget to consider soft X-rays as a culprit.

## Summary and outlook

Compared to the temperatures generated by a laser microbeam, the surface of the Sun is a cool place indeed in the Universe. But the duration of a microbeam inferno is only a few nanoseconds. This will have (positive) consequences for work with biological matter. The next section will address this perspective.

## 2.2 Interaction of pulsed lasers with biological matter

The previous sections have shown us that extremely high intensities and temperatures can be generated with comparatively small laser powers. We have now available intensities ranging from very small (which we can achieve simply by attenuation of the beam or by running the laser with less than maximum power) up to the extreme values calculated in the previous section.

It is almost trivial to state that the mechanism of interaction with tissue depends on intensity. In order to learn in detail how different ranges of intensity interact with tissue, we can draw on the experience of laser diagnostics in the range of small intensities, and the experience of medicine in the intermediate and high intensity range (Boxes 16 and 17). For very high intensities, which so far have never been used in biological and biomedical applications, we have to do our own estimates. Information from protein folding studies will help us to gain some idea about the possible interaction of the extreme intensities and temperatures (Section 2.2.3). Finally, in Section 2.2.4, we will discuss one of the most startling properties of laser microtools: the fact that one can work in the interior of an object without opening it.

### 2.2.1 High intensities in medical surgery

The effects of laser tissue interactions are well studied in the context of medical laser surgery which uses the whole intensity range except the upper extreme values. In Box 16 some "medical" laser types and their primary field of applications are listed.

Laser techniques can provide a wide range of medical effects, from slight heating in biostimulation to coagulation to plasma generation. Since in most medical applications large amounts of tissue have to be treated the lasers cannot be focused to the extreme precision as in laser microbeams.

The spatial accuracy required in medical laser surgery is of the order of a few hundred micrometers, i.e. focusing a medical laser is comparably simple and lenses or objectives with small numerical apertures can be used. The focus of such optical elements can range from several millimeters up to many centimeters. The working distance is large and thus it is possible to operate conveniently.

**Box 16: Typical applications of different lasers in medicine**

| Laser type | Wavelength (nm) | Typical applications |
|---|---|---|
| Excimer 308 | | Correction of eye lens errors (cornea shaping) opening of clotted arteries (removal of stenoses) dentistry |
| Argon ion | 514.4 | Sealing the retina to the eye's choroid |
| NdYAG | 532 | Same as argon ion lasers, He-Ne lasers |
| He-Ne | 621 | Biostimulation |
| NdYAG | 1064 | Coagulation, tissue melting, internal heat application |
| Holmium YAG | 2120 | Same as NdYAG |
| Erbium YAG | 2936 | Same as excimer lasers, but can be transported better by light guides |
| $CO_2$ | 10600 | Cutting, welding, drilling holes; standard laser of medical surgery |
| Dye | variable | Experimental |

**Box 17: Interaction of light of varying intensity with matter**

| Intensity | Type of interaction | Mechanism of interaction | Application |
|---|---|---|---|
| $mW/cm^2$ | Biostimulation | Influence on certain elements of metabolism | Stimulation of wound healing |
| $KW/cm^2$ | Coagulation | Denaturation and fixation of tissue | Sealing of tissue |
| $MW/cm^2$ | Evaporation | Water boils off tissue disintegrates | Tissue incision |
| $GW/cm^2$ | Photoablation, Photodisruption | Single molecular bonds break | Eruptive ablation of tissue |
| $TW/cm^2$ | Microplasms | Molecules are totally destroyed | Working regime of a good laser microbeam |

One has to pay a price for this convenience: In order to reach, for example, an intensity of $3 \cdot 10^6$ W/cm$^2$ which is less than a 100 mW NdYAG laser can generate and orders of magnitude below the comparably small nitrogen laser in laser microtools, one has to use a 1 kilowatt laser focused to a diameter of 200 micrometers. 1 kilowatt means that each second 1 kilojoule energy is deposited into the tissue. This large amount of energy causes secondary damage and, in fact, carbonisation of healthy surrounding tissue during medical laser surgery is often considered to be a serious problem.

## 2.2.2 Photons cooperate at extreme intensities

Here we need to take a short excursion back to basic physics (Section 1.1.1). When we calculate for a medical laser or a laser microbeam how many photons occupy the same space we will end up with tens of thousand or more (if you want to verify this, use the type of calculations shown in Box 3).

Due to their "social" behavior (Section 1.1.3) the photons can cooperate with each other and simulate the effects of light with shorter wavelengths due to two-, three-... photon effects. At the highest intensities (although not so much in medical surgery) almost all wavelengths can be simulated and for interactions it is of primary importance what heat is generated and what electrical fields prevail. In principle, the absorption coefficient of a material at a given wavelength should be irrelevant. Due to a complex interplay of the light with the tissue in the very first instants of interaction, this is only partly true. Wavelength still plays a role, but in combination with the intensity effects. We will learn in Section 2.3 that for small and intermediate intensities the situation is completely different. A special case of multiphoton effects are two-photon effects. The latter are discussed in some detail in Appendix A5.

## 2.2.3 Heat shocks from a laser microbeam: Too fast to damage proteins

At first glance it appears strange that extreme physical conditions can be used in biology and medicine. What happens to biological tissue when it is locally heated by 100 000 degrees or more? At sites where the laser hits directly, physical plasma will be generated. Chemical bonds will break. No molecules will survive. But all this happens in a spot focused to below 0.5 micrometer. What happens in the vicinity of this spot?

You have already learned that the extreme heat is decreased to almost room temperature within a few tens of nanoseconds (Box 14, previous chapter). What does such a short, though extreme, heat shock mean for biological tissue? Experimental data are rare since it is difficult to measure such short processes. But at least for protein molecules we have some information, partially from folding studies, partially directly from unfolding experiments. For example, pentapeptides can fold within nanoseconds (Tobias et al., 1991). The small protein "Barstar" refolds with submillisecond speed after a heat shock from 2 to 10 degrees centigrade (Nölting et al., 1995). Also, the reaction of the protein apomyoglobin can be studied on such a short time scale by Raman spectroscopy. A peak in the Raman spectrum of apomyoglobin called amide I band gives information on the structural state of the protein's backbone. When apomyoglobin is heated by 60 °C with the help of a pulse from a YAG pumped dye laser (3 mJ, wavelength 1.9 mm, focused to 200 mm diameter) it is slighty denatured but folds reversibly back into its native form with a relaxation time of 40 ns. Since the process is totally reversible, one can assume that the denaturation (in which we are interested) is slower than refolding. The duration of the heat shock itself (Box 14), however, is shorter. As a result we have reason to believe that the heat wave is faster than the denaturation process.

An even more detailed study exists for the 21 amino acid long model peptide (Williams et al., 1996, Gilmanshin et al., 1997):

$$Suc-A5-(AAARA)_3A-NH_2$$

where A is Alanine and R is Arginine.

It tends to form an alpha-helix which is denatured by heat. A laser induced temperature jump from 18 to 46 degrees centigrade causes unfolding with a time constant of $160 \pm 60$ ns. The refolding has a time constant of 16 ns. There is no overall denaturation of the peptide at 46 degrees centigrade. With the assumption that the unfolding step doubles with every 10 degrees centigrade while the folding step remains unaffected (the latter is unreasonable but leaves us on the safe side), even at close to 100 degrees centigrade there is no overall denaturation by laser pulses with a duration of a few tens of nanoseconds.

In total it can be concluded that the phase of high temperature is too short to thermally cause significant secondary damage. There may, however, be some photodamage caused by scattered light. Fortunately we do not have to rely solely on theoretical estimates. Experiments will confirm that laser microbeams work with high precision. Particularly in the context of laser microdissection of chromosomes (Section 5.4.2) we will investigate secondary damage by electron microscopy and find out that it is small.

## 2.2.4 Working in the interior of closed objects

We will now address the question of why it is possible to work in the interior of closed objects. This is possible since we work with high apertures, i.e. that the lasers are focused very sharply. In case you wish to know more about numerical apertures you refer to Appendix A2.7 or, for practical aspects, to Box 8 of Section 1.3.6. Fig. 16 shows the principle.

Let us discuss the case of a numerical aperture of 1 when using a dry objective, i.e. when working in air, without any liquid between the objective and object. Let us assume a diameter of the outermost objective lens of 200 mm as well as a working length of 200 mm (approximately such values are found for 100x objectives). Let us assume that the intensity (power density) at the objective is $I_o$. The light is focused into a cone. At half way from the objective to the object plane, the diameter of this cone is half of that at the objective, i.e. the intensity is four times of that at the objective. At a distance of x mm from the focus the intensity I(x) is

$$I(x) = Io \cdot (200/x)^2. \quad (24)$$

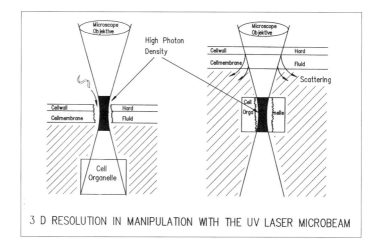

3 D RESOLUTION IN MANIPULATION WITH THE UV LASER MICROBEAM

**Fig. 16:** Working in the interior of an unopened object. The focus can be directed toward the cell wall, to an intracellular organelle of the nucleus. At a certain distance from the point of focus the intensity is sufficiently small (see Box 18) so as not to damage other parts of the cell.

Due to diffraction the intensity of the focused laser beam does not further increase at distances closer than approx. 0.5 μm from the geometric focus. Therefore, this power density is assumed to be the power density in the focus. Box 18 gives some quantitative values.

**Box 18: Relative intensity at different distances from the laser focus**

| x | $I(x)/I_o$ |
|---|---|
| 0.5 μm | 100 % |
| 1 μm | 25 % |
| 2 μm | 6 % |
| 5 μm | 1 % |
| 10 μm | 0.25 % |

When working in the center of a comparably small spherical cell with 10 μm diameter the cell surface is 5 μm apart from the focus. There, the intensity is only 1% of that in the focus. In other words: an intensity Io can be found for which one can work on subcellular structures of a cell while the cell's surface is not severely damaged. Things become even more pronounced with larger cells, such as cells from plants which often have diameters of several tens of micrometers.

One can calculate similarly that the intensity decreases much less at lower numerical apertures. Thus it is clear that working in the depth of unopened cells is only possible with numerical apertures close to 1 (ideally above 1).

With a nitrogen laser we had already calculated a maximum intensity of approximately $10^{13}$ W per cm² in the focus. At the cell surface (5 μm away) this is still $10^{11}$ Watt per/cm² which might still damage the cell membrane, therefore, in order to use the microbeam inside an unopened cell one has to reduce the power. In real experiments this is done by trial and error i.e. test cells are treated with the laser microbeam until an attenuation for the laser is found where damage at the cell surface is no longer observed.

## Summary and outlook

Short pulsed and highly focused lasers allow precise micromachining even inside closed objects. It is not so much the wavelength but the intensity which governs the mechanisms of interaction with biological matter. Continuous lasers, which are the basis for optical tweezers, are very different.

**Selected literature:**

B. Nölting, R. Golbik and A.R. Fersht (1995) Submillisecond events in protein folding. Proc. Natl. Acad. Sci 92.23, 10668-10672.

D.J. Tobias, J.E. Mertz and C.L. Brooks (1995) Nanosecond time scale folding dynamics of a pentapeptide in water. Biochemistry 30, 6054-6058.

S. Williams, T.P. Casagrove, R. Gilmanshin, K.S. Fang R.H. Callendar, W.H. Woodroff and R.B. Dyer (1996) Fast events in protein folding; Helix melting and formation in a small peptide. Biochemistry 35, 690-697.

R. Gilmanshin, S. Williams, R.H. Callender, W.H. Woodruff and R.B. Dyer (1997) Fast events in protein folding: Relaxation dynamics of secondary and tertiary structure in native apomyoglobin. Proc. Natl. Acad. Sci. 94, 3709-3713.

# 2.3 Interaction of optical tweezers with biological material

Continuous wave (cw) lasers often provide higher average powers (measured, for example, as the energy generated over several seconds) than pulsed lasers. There is, however, no such thing as a peak power. In other words: The average power is identical with the maximum power. The intensities generated by cw lasers are usually not sufficient to generate multiphoton effects. Therefore, in contrast to focused pulsed lasers, the working wavelength of cw lasers is important for the effects which can be generated.

## 2.3.1 The wavelength makes the difference

The major hazard to biological material manipulated by lasers is damage caused by absorption and heating. In some cases such an effect is in fact desired, for example, in experiments where chromosomes in living cells are severed and subsequently the effects of such invasion on cell behavior can be observed (see Section

4.2). Particularly in optical trapping experiments one would like to make use solely of the forces generated by scattering of light. In such cases, absorption is an unwanted side effect and should be minimized.

In order to describe absorption of light by tissue, the Lambert Beer law can be used (see Appendix A5)

$$I(x) = I_o \cdot \exp(-\varepsilon \cdot c \cdot x). \quad (25)$$

When light penetrates a tissue it is attenuated. In the depth $x=1/\varepsilon \cdot c$ the argument of the exponential function in equation 25 is -1. Since $\exp(-1)=1/e$ or $1/2.71$ we obtain

$$I(x_p) = I_o/e. \quad (26)$$

Unfortunately, in tissue this cannot be used to calculate a molar extinction coefficient $\varepsilon$, since the concentration c of absorbing molecules is not known. Therefore the product $\varepsilon \cdot c$ has to be treated as one single mathematical value. It is called the penetration depth. It is the thickness of the tissue layer, after which the original light intensity has decreased to 36.9% (=1/e, =1/2.71).

In tissue, absorption and therefore the penetration depth is dependent on wavelength, since a tissue is a mixture of a wide variety of molecules. The following rules of thumb are valid in a first approximation:

- In the ultraviolet range DNA (around 260 nm) and proteins (280–300 nm) are the major absorbers. UV absorption is similar for many types of tissue.
- At visible wavelengths there can be numerous absorbing agents (flavins, chlorophyll, hemoglobin, NAD, NADH). Here absorption is highly tissue-specific and is, for example, responsible for the color of tissues.
- At infrared wavelengths, the absorption of biological material is governed by the absorption of water. This is low around 1000 nm and increases to high values for wavelengths approaching 3000 nm.

The quantitative variations with wavelengths are dramatic. Box 19 gives values for a typical tissue and laser wavelengths typical for laser surgery and microtools.

Box 19 may serve as a first guide to judge which type of laser is suitable for a given task. For example, ultraviolet lasers are highly absorbed and therefore the light sources of choice for ablation studies. In turn, NdYAG lasers are ideally suited for optical trapping. Visible lasers may serve both purposes, but low efficiency in ablation studies or significant absorption in trapping studies prevent optimization of their performance.

**Box 19: Penetration depth for the working wavelengths of different lasers**

| Wavelength (nm) and laser | Penetration depth (mm) |
|---|---|
| 193 (ArF excimer laser) | 1 |
| 308 (XeCl excimer laser) | 50 |
| 337 (nitrogen) | 60 |
| 550 (visible laser) | *) |
| 1064 (NdYAG) | 1000 |
| 2120 (HoYAG) | 420 |
| 2940 (Er:YAG) | 1 |
| 10600 ($CO_2$) | 12 |

*) The penetration depth at visible wavelengths (400–800 nm) depends highly on the specific properties of the material. The values in the infrared range are simply the inverse absorption coefficients of water. In the ultraviolet range, data of Welch et al., 1991 have been used. See also Furzikov, 1987.

## 2.3.2 Thermal effects in continuous laser microbeams

Heat generation caused by absorption of laser light is governed by several counteracting processes:
1. Only the absorbed energy can be converted into heat.
2. Often, part of the energy is used up for bond cleavage and other photochemical processes.
3. During absorption the generated heat starts to flow into the environment. When a cw laser is used, an equilibrium between heating and flow of heat will govern the process. Material constants such as thermal conductivity will be relevant.

The amount of absorbed energy can be calculated when the penetration depth of a given laser wavelength is known. The order of magnitude of energy used for photochemical processes can at least be estimated. The problem is to calculate the heat flow.

Several formulas exist to quantify thermal effects. They have been developed for the processing of non-living solid-state materials, which absorb practically all of the incident laser light and transform almost all of the absorbed energy into heat. The temperature increase T induced on a solid state material by a continuous laser can be calculated as

$$T = (1-R)\cdot W/(\pi\cdot r\cdot K) \quad (27)$$

where R is the reflectivity of the material, W is the laser power, r is the beam radius and K is the thermal conductivity.

**Box 20: Thermal conductivities for some selected materials:**

| Material | K in W/(cm·°C) |
|---|---|
| Diamond | 330 |
| Silver | 4.27 |
| Aluminium | 2.37 |
| Water | 0.00059 |

For example, in fully absorbing aluminium a 1 kilowatt laser with a radius of 0.1 cm will cause a temperature increase of

$$T = 10^3 \text{ W}/(\pi\cdot 0.1 \text{ cm} \cdot 2.4 \text{ W/cm}\cdot^\circ\text{C}) \quad (28)$$

$$T = 1330 \text{ }^\circ\text{C}$$

or 1.33°C per watt.

Somewhat more difficult is to calculate the temperature rise in transparent biological material since it is difficult to estimate how much of the light is absorbed. This problem can be solved experimentally as described below.

### 2.3.3 Interaction of NdYAG optical tweezers (1064 nm) with cells

Liu et al. (1995) have measured these data for a model liposome of 10 μm diameter and for ovary cells from Chinese hamster (CHO) cells.

For such a measurement a fluorescent dye with temperature-dependent emission spectrum is suitable. The dye used in these experiments has the common name laurdan (chemically: 6-dodecanoyl-2-dimethyl-amino-anaphthalene). It can be embedded in artificial membranes (phospholipid bilayers) or in natural cell membranes. Between 28 and 38 degrees centigrade the fluorescence emission maximum shifts from less than 450 nm to more than 480 nm. Such a shift can be measured with good accuracy. More on laurdan will be discussed in the section on two-photon effects (2.3.5)

The liposome or the cell were held by different powers of NdYAG optical tweezers, focused to a micrometer. The powers were measured in the object plane. The temperature in the membranes was measured on the basis of the fluorescence spectra of embedded laurdan. The result was

$$1.45 \pm 0.15 \ °C/100 \ mW \text{ for the liposome}$$
$$1.15 \pm 0.25 \ °C/100 \ mW \text{ for the CHO cell.}$$

Both values are only valid with good accuracy up to 250 mW, but for crude estimates they can certainly be used up to considerably higher values. Since the lasers were focused to a diameter of approximately 1 µm (corresponding to a cross sectional area of $10^{-8} \ cm^2$), a good rule of thumb is

$$1.25 \ °C \text{ per } 10^7 \ W/cm^2 \text{ (for 1064 nm).}$$

## 2.3.4 The surprise: NdYAG lasers are not the best choice

A direct comparison of a NdYAG laser with a Ti Sapphire laser tunable from 700 nm to 1000 nm showed qualitatively that the latter is better suited for optical trapping than NdYAG lasers (Berns et al., 1992).

While Box 19 and the result obtained above indicate that near infrared wavelengths are better suited for optical trapping than other wavelengths, the final test of suitability of a given wavelength for optical trapping can only come from an experiment testing the viability. Perhaps the most convincing proof of viability is cell division and the generation of healthy progeny. On a single-cell basis this can be tested in a cloning assay where an individual cell is transferred in a microreaction vessel with cell medium and allowed to divide. Such a study has been performed by Liang et al. (1996).

Cells from the ovary of a Chinese hamster (CHO cells) were optically trapped at laser powers in the object plane of 58 mW and 176 mW (corresponding to 26 and 52 MW/cm$^2$). The duration of trapping ranged from less than a minute to up to 20 minutes. Two types of lasers were tested: a NdYAG laser at 1064 nm and a tunable continuous wave titanium sapphire laser generating wavelengths from 700 to 990 nm.

After trapping, the CHO cells were transferred into the culture vessel and allowed to divide for 5 to 6 days. When approximately 50 healthy looking cells were counted the cell was rated "clonable." Several control experiments were performed, including one where cells were cells in the microscope but not illuminated by lasers. Their clonability was set at 100%. For cells trapped in the laser the clonability decreased with increasing trapping time and increasing power density.

These results were much as one would have expected. The surprise came when the wavelength was varied. The wavelength dependence showed a highly peaked structure, i.e. the viability (clonability) of the CHO cells depends very specifically on the wavelength. For example, after 3 minutes of trapping the following results were obtained:

1. The least damage occurred at 960 nm (almost 100% clonability) and at 830 nm (90%). Also, at wavelengths below 750 nm the clonability appears to increase towards visible wavelengths, but the study did not cover this range completely.
2. Relative minima in clonability after 3-minute trapping were found at 900 nm (60% clonability) and at 760 nm (a few percent). The clonability after three minutes trapping with the traditional trapping wavelength of 1064 nm was also only 60%. For longer trapping times, 1064 nm are even more damaging: After 10 minutes the cloning efficiency drops to 20%, almost as low as in the minima at 900 nm and 760 nm.

Strictly, these data apply only to the CHO cells. However, they are, at least in their basic message, confirmed by an earlier study on the formation of abnormal chromosome bridges after optical trapping (Vorobjev, 1993). It remains interesting to see how far these studies can be generalized and how far the clonability increases when the study is extended towards visible wavelengths, before specific absorption takes over and completely severs cells.

## 2.3.5 Two-photon excited fluorescence for detecting damage in IR optical traps

The cloning assay gives very clear information on cell damage but it is difficult to perform. A simpler way to assess damage entails the use of suitable fluorescence dyes with specific properties distinguishing healthy from damaged or dead cells. The following dyes are particularly useful:

- *Laurdan*: It has been already referred to in section 2.3.3 in the context of temperature measurements. It is also sensitive for membrane fluidity and polarity.
- The dye pair *SYBR14/Propidium iodide*: SYBR14 fluorescence green, propidium iodide red. The pair can be used to distinguish live from dead cells since viable cells incorporate SYBR 14 and appear green while dead cells incorporate propidium iodide as well and then appear red.
- *Rhodamine 123*: acts as a marker for mitochondrial activity
- *Acridine orange:* detects single strand breaks.
- The natural coenzymes *NADH* and *NADPH*: Are present in all cells; can be employed as bioindicators of metabolic function (autofluorescence).

Usually all these dyes are excited by visible or UV wavelengths. Laurdan, for example, is a dye used in two-photon microscopy. Even three-photon excitation is possible and has been studied in detail for the fluorescent dye indo 1 (Szymacinski, 1996 and Yu et al., 1996). For more details on two- or three-photon effects see Appendix section A5.4.

Exploiting two-photon excitation the infrared trapping wavelengths of 760 nm and 800 nm (both not visible) can also excite fluorescence and thus the same laser can be used to trap cells and visualize the effects of trapping by two-photon fluorescence excitation. At least occasionally two photons will occupy the same volume element. In addition, experience from spectroscopy shows that at $10 \, MW/cm^2$, i.e. at power densities typical for optical trapping, these two photon effects can constitute the majority of interactions.

A number of studies of this type have been performed (see list of selected literature). For example, two-photon fluorescence excitation was used to induce visible fluorescence in sperm cells trapped with 760 nm and with 800 nm. The following set of results has been obtained (Liu et al., 1995; König et al., 1995):

1. In the two-photon excited autofluorescence due to NADH/NADPH) the intensity increased up to 100-fold upon trapping with 760 nm for 10 min but not with trapping at 800 nm.
2. In xenofluorescence studies with the live/dead dye pair fluorescence changed from green to red after half a minute indicating cell death. Simultaneously flagellar motion of the sperm cells ceased and the cloning assay described in the wavelength studies did no longer yield clones.

In these experiments the two-photon effect has only been used to *excite fluorescence* by the infrared trapping laser, while the damage is obviously induced by single-photon effects. In an early experiment multiphoton effects obviously *caused damage*. An effect called "phase paling" is known to be induced by short UV wavelengths. Calmettes (1983) reported that they found phase paling in chromosomes and nucleoli from rat kangaroo kidney cells after irradiation with 532 nm and 266 nm from a frequency-doubled and -quadrupled NdYAG laser. They interpreted their results as two- and four-photon effects.

## Summary and outlook

The best lasers for optical tweezers have working wavelengths in the near infrared region, below 1100 nm. Absorption of these wavelengths by tissue is minimal and therefore light pressure and gradient forces can be exploited optimally. As a rule of thumb, a continuous 100 mW NdYAG laser heats biological tissue up by 1 to 1.5 degrees.

## Selected literature

M.W. Berns, J.B. Aist, W.H. Wright and H. Liang (1992) Optical trapping in animal and fungal cells using a tunable near-infrared titanium-sapphire laser. Exp. Cell. Res. 188, 375-378.

P.P. Calmettes and M.W. Berns (1983) Laser-induced mutiphoton processes in living cells. Proc. Natl. Acad. Sci. 80, 7197-7199.

N.P. Furzikov (1987) Different lasers for angioplasty: Thermo optical comparison. IEEE J. Quant. Elect. QE 23, 1751-1755.

K. König, H. Liang, M.W. Berns and B.J. Tromberg (1995) Cell damage by near-IR microbeams. Nature 377, 20-21.

H. Liang, K. Tong, T. Ching Trang, D. Shin, S. Kimel and M.W. Berns (1996) Wavelength dependence of cell cloning efficiency after optical trapping. Bioph. J. 70, 1-5.

Y. Liu, D.K. Cheng, G.J. Sonek, M.W. Berns, C.F. Chapman and B.J. Tromberg (1995) Evidence for localized cell heating induced by IR optical tweezers. Bioph. J. 68.5, 2137-2144.

Y. Liu, G.J. Sonek, M.W. Berns, K. König and B.J. Tromberg (1995) Two-photon fluorescence excitation in continuous-wave infrared optical tweezers. Applied Optics 20, 2246-2248.

H. Szymacinski, I. Gryczynski and J.R. Lakowicz (1996) Three-photon induced fluorescence of the calcium probe indo 1. Bioph. J. 70, 547-555.

I.A. Vorobjev, H. Liang, W.H. Wright and M.W. Berns (1993) Optical trapping for chromosome manipulation: a wavelength dependence of induced chromosome bridges. Bioph. J. 64, 533-538.

A.J. Welch, M. Motamedi, S. Rastegar, G.L. Le Carpentier and D. Jansen (1991) Laser thermal ablation. Photochemistry and Photobiology 53, 815-823.

W. Yu, P.T.C. So, T. French and E. Gratton (1996) Fluorescence generalized polarization of cell membranes: A two photon scanning microscopy approach. Bioph. J. 70, 626-636.

## 2.4 Light pressure: Some quantitative relationships

### 2.4.1 Calculating some surprising facts

While the effects of heat are probably familiar to you from the use of laser light in industrial processes, the fact that light exerts pressure is often regarded as an exotic textbook curiosity with no practical use. But you already know that this is not correct and in the introductory chapters you have already learned a first simple formula for the calculation of light pressure and light force from the intensity of a laser beam. The following chapters will show you how one can calculate light pressure quantitatively. Perhaps you will again be surprised about the magnitude of the effects one can achieve with light.

### Box 21: Kiloponds and kilograms in everyday language

A weight can be measured in kiloponds or newtons (10 N=1 kp, see also Box 1).

At the surface of the Earth a mass of 1 kg exerts a force of 1 kp.

Only there is a kilopond equivalent to a kilogram. On the moon, 1 kg exerts a force of approx. 1/6 kp.

In everyday language often kg and kp are confused; i.e., one says that an object has a weight of ... kilograms.

You should keep this in mind for the following discussion.

The underlying physical equation is

$$force = mass \cdot acceleration$$
$$or\ acceleration = force/mass$$

which was already discussed in Box 2 of Section 1.1.2.

The effects of light pressure are quite small in daily life. For example, a car in sunlight is less than a millipond heavier than in the shade. The force which is exerted on the planet Earth by sunlight corresponds to a mass of ten thousand tons at the Earth's surface, large but not dramatic for such a big object. When a continuous laser with moderate power of one Watt is focused to the diffraction limit, it can exert a force of approximately 5 nanonewton, again, not very much. Two billion times this force corresponds to 1 kilopond.

But microscopic objects have very small masses which can be accelerated dramatically even by small forces. An object, which can just be illuminated with such a focused laser, however, is also very small. For example, a bacterium with a diameter of 1 μm has a weight of approximately one picogram only. By a force of 5 nanonewton it is accelerated with 30000-fold gravitational acceleration, comparable to the acceleration in an ultracentrifuge. Since the distances over which acceleration can occur are only short, it does not mean that microscopic particles can be accelerated to very high speeds. It means rather that they can be moved against quite strong viscous forces over a comparatively short distance. If you wish to know in detail how theses values can be calculated, refer to Boxes 22–24.

## Box 22: Light pressure and forces on a car in the sun

Here it is shown that the pressure exerted by sunlight increases the weight of a car.
It is assumed that the car has a surface area of 5 m².
In a first step the dimension W/m² of the intensity of sunlight at the Earth's surface
$(1.35 \cdot 10^3$ W/m²) is converted into a suitable form. We use 1 W=1 J/s
and 1 J=1 Nm (see Box 1 of Section 1.1.2)

$$W = 1.35 \cdot 10^3 \ Wm^2$$

$$W = 1.35 \cdot 10^3 \ J/s/m^2$$

$$W = 1.35 \cdot 10^3 \ Nm/s/m^2$$

Now we insert the latter form into Equation (13) of Section 1.1.5: P= I/c where
c=3·10⁸ m/s

$$P = \frac{1.35 \cdot 10^3}{3 \cdot 10^8} \frac{(Nm/s)/m^2}{m/s}$$

$$P = 0.45 \cdot 10^{-5} \ N/m^2$$

The force defined as pressure·area
$$F = 0.45 \cdot 10^{-5} \ N/m^2 \cdot 5 \ m^2$$

$$F = 2.25 \cdot 10^{-6} \ N$$

$$F = 0.225 \cdot 10^{-6} \ kp$$

and this corresponds to approx. 0.2 milligram at the Earth's surface.

## Box 23: Sunlight on the planet Earth: Some ten thousand tons

The cross sectional area of the Earth is approx. $115 \cdot 10^{12}$ m². It is hit by the same intensity as the car in Box 17, i.e. the light pressure force acting on the Earth is

$$0.45 \cdot 10^{-5} \ N/m^2 \cdot 115 \cdot 10^{12} \ m^2 \approx 50000 \ kilopond.$$

This is the force which a mass of 50000 tons would exert on the Earth' s surface.

**Box 24: Acceleration of a microscopic object by a 1 Watt laser**

The force which is exerted by a 1 Watt laser can be directly calculated in analogy to example 1 but it is best to use equation 12 of Section 1.1.5, F=W/c

$$F = \frac{1 Nm/s}{3 \cdot 10^8 \ m/s}$$

$$F = 3.3 \cdot 10^{-9} \ N = 3.3 \ nanonewton$$

When this radiation is focused, for example, onto a bacterium with a volume of 1 femtoliter or a mass of 1 picogram, it will accelerate it over a short distance.

Using $1 \ N = 10^5 \ gcm/s^2$) one obtains with the equation of Box 16:

$$acceleration = \frac{3.3 \cdot 10^{-9}}{10^{-12}} \ \frac{N}{g} = \frac{3.3 \cdot 10^{-4}}{10^{-12}} \ \frac{gcm/s^2}{g}$$

$$acceleration = 3.3 \cdot 10^8 \ cm/s^2$$

$$acceleration = 3.3 \cdot 10^6 \ m/s^2$$

$$acceleration = 330000 \ gravitational \ accelerations$$

## 2.4.2 Mie particles: The color of the target affects the light force

You may have noticed that Box 21 showed how to calculate the force acting on a *black* car. Indeed, the force is dependent on the color of the target. Why?

The answer is surprisingly simple. In this example the target was much larger than the wavelength of light. Such objects are called Mie particles. For such targets one can think in simple terms of absorption or reflection. In some ways they act as a sort of mirror. The whole light wave impinges onto the object and its whole momentum can be transferred to the target. For fully reflecting targets (silver is ideal, white is a good approximation) the momentum transfer is twice as large. Any situation between these two extremes is also possible for other colors. This is occasionally allowed for by introducing a dimensionless factor g into Equations 14 and 15 in Section 1.1.5 whose value ranges from 1 to 2. Unless stated otherwise we will neglect the factor, i.e. we will assume that the target is black.

## 2.4.3 Light forces on very small (Rayleigh) particles

In the other extreme, particles are much smaller than the wavelength of the used light. Such particles, often molecules or macromolecular complexes, are called Rayleigh particles. They act like antenna. Generally it is thought that antenna should have at least the size of half the wavelength. However, even much smaller objects can interact with electromagnetic waves of a given wavelength – albeit with highly reduced efficiency. The basic difference to Mie scattering is that the light is neither absorbed nor reflected, but scattered elastically. The transferred momentum and the resulting force is related to the change in momentum of the light. Thus, not the incident power but the scattered power is relevant for a quantitative description of Rayleigh scattering. The theory of Rayleigh scattering quantifies this process on the basis of electrodynamics. The derivation is somewhat bulky. If you want to go into more detail refer to Boxes 24 and 25 or to Appendix A5. In its most simple version, the light pressure acting on a Rayleigh particle is

$$P = 4148 \cdot r'^4 \cdot R \cdot I/c. \quad (29)$$

This looks pretty much like the formula for Mie scattering except that some factors are added. $r'$ is the ratio of the particle's true diameter divided by the wavelength. R represents (but is not identical to) the refractive index of the particle in water. For most particles R is between 0 and 1 (see Box 26). Since the formula is valid only for $r' < 0.1$, the product of all numerical factors is smaller than 1, i.e.

$$P < I/c. \quad (30)$$

From this you can see that light pressure on Rayleigh particles is smaller than on Mie particles.

## Box 25: Light pressure for Rayleigh particles

The *scattered* portion of the total power is given as (see Appendix A5)

$$W_{scat} = I \cdot (128 \ \pi^5 r^6/3 \ \lambda^4) \cdot ((n^2-1)/(n^2+2))^2$$

where r is the radius of the Rayleigh particle, I the wavelength and n is the refractive index of the particle. The force which light of power W exerts on Rayleigh particles is then

$$F_{scat} = I/c \cdot ((128 \ \pi^5 r^6/3 \ \lambda^4) \cdot n_1 \cdot ((n^2-1)/(n^2+2))^2)$$

At a first glance it may be confusing to encounter an expression I/c, which occurs above in the equation for light pressure rather than in the equation for the force. The reason for this is that the area of the Rayleigh particle, $r^2\pi$ is hidden in the other factors. In order to calculate the pressure, one has just to divide the force equation by the area

$$P_{scat} = I/c \cdot ((128 \ \pi^4 r^4/3 \ \lambda^4) \cdot n_1 \cdot ((n^2-1)/(n^2+2))^2).$$


## Box 26: Simplifying the light pressure equation for Rayleigh particles

When all quantities in Box 25 containing refractive indices are put into the refractive index factor R

$$R = n_1 \cdot ((n^2-1)/(n^2+2))^2$$

and with $r'=r/\lambda$ , the equation for the light pressure becomes

$$P_{scat} = 4148 \cdot r'^4 \cdot R \cdot I/c$$

where the numerical factor has just collected all dimensionless quantities. $4148 \cdot r'^4$ is approximately 1 for r'=1/8, but becomes rapidly smaller for smaller particles. In turn, for larger particles the Rayleigh theory becomes increasingly inaccurate.

The refractive index factor is also smaller than 1. Some typical refractive index factors in water ($n_1$=1.3345) for different refractive indices n of the target are:

| n | R |
|------|------|
| 1.0 | 0 |
| 1.5 | 0.39 |
| 2.0 | 0.66 |
| 3.0 | 0.97 |

## Summary and outlook

Light exerts pressure in the direction of its own propagation. There is a difference for particles whose wavelength is small as compared to the wavelength of light (Rayleigh particles) and for large particles. Light pressure can be used to accelerate objects or to balance them, for example, against gravity. This is the reason why comet tails are always directed away from the sun. When the sun is shining on a car, one can measure this with a balance with an accuracy of a few milliponds. When a continuous laser is focused to its theoretical limit, the acceleration of the corresponding volume element is comparable to accelerations in an ultracentrifuge.

# 2.5 Gradient forces: Full control in three dimensions

With light pressure one can buoy microscopic objects against the force of gravity, similarly as a ping pong ball can be balanced on a fountain of water. Such an interplay of forces is not exactly what one needs to fix microscopic objects in three dimensions. An additional effect makes life even simpler: A laser beam with higher intensity at the optical axis than in the periphery drives a sphere with suitable properties (see below) towards the optical axis. Moreover, when highly focused laser light is used, conditions can be found under which such a sphere is pulled into the focus even against the action of light pressure. Incredible? Impossible? No, in fact this is surprisingly simple to understand! In some ways this process is comparable to a boat sailing against the wind.

### 2.5.1 Axial and transversal effects

These forces are called gradient forces. A particle has to be dielectric in order to feel gradient forces. To be dielectric means that electric dipoles can be induced. Metal spheres are not dielectric. Plastic spheres and biological cells are. In terms of optics, something is dielectric not if it reflects, but if it refracts light. Therefore, gradient forces are, for example, dependent on the refractive indices of the object and of the medium. Additionally they are dependent on the beam quality of the focused light. Since so far nobody has found a way to calculate such forces precisely, one usually quantifies gradient forces semiempirically. A quality factor Q is introduced into Equations 12 or 13 of Section 1.1.5 which then become

$$F = Q \cdot W/c \quad (31)$$

and

$$P = Q \cdot I/c. \quad (32)$$

### Box 27: Experimental (axial and transversal) Q values for various sphere sizes and materials and for different focusing

For practical work, Wright et al. (1994) have determined Q values for different experimental situations. In that publication axial forces generated by an NdYAG laser (1064 nm) against the direction of light propagation (axial backward forces) and forces perpendicular to this direction (transverse forces) have been calculated and measured.

The table below summarizes the major results for different sphere sizes, numerical apertures of the microscope objectives and different polarizations of the lasers. For transversal forces one has to consider that laser light is polarized. As one can see for the transversal effects from the left side of table, it makes a difference if the polarization is also transversal or if it is perpendicular to it.

Percentage (100·Q) for different experiments and theoretical predictions (in brackets)

| Type of force | Axial | Axial | Transversal | Transversal | Transversal |
|---|---|---|---|---|---|
| Numerical aperture | 1.25 -1.3 | 0.8 | 1.3 | 1.3 | 0.8 |
| Polarization | | | Parallel | Perpendic | Perpendic |
| 1 µm Silica | 0.4–0.6% | | 15% (16%) | 13% (15%) | |
| 5 µm Polystyrene | 7% | | 21% (36%) | 19% (29%) | |
| 10 µm Polystyrene | 2.8–8.4% | 1.3–1.4% | 37% (36%) | 29% (29%) | |
| 20 µm Polystyrene | 10% | | 41% (36%) | 32% (29%) | 28% (13%) |
| Remark: | Low values: far from cover glass; high values: close to cover glass | | In brackets: theoretical values predicted by electromagnetic theory for the 1 µm sphere and by ray optics for the larger ones | | |

There are several detailed studies available where the value of Q is determined for different experimental situations (for example, Wright, 1994). Gradient forces can act axially, i.e. against the direction of light propagation and perpendicularly to it. Both forces can cooperate to pull an object against light pressure into the focus. For

1 μm silica microbeads, the axial value for Q is of the order of 0.05 (or 5%), the transversal value is approximately 15% of the value for pure light pressure, for which Q is by definition =1 corresponding to 100%). The values for 20 μm poly-styrene microbeads are 0.1 and up to 0.4, i.e. 10% and up to 40% of the light pressure value. For more details see Box 27.

As a rule of thumb, one can say that gradient forces of optimally focused light pull an object into the focus with a force corresponding to a few percent of the force which one would calculate using the simple light force formula. The lateral light forces can amount to up to 40%

In Section 2.5.2 you will find a simple explanation why parallel light stabilizes refracting spheres on the optical axis and Section 2.5.3 will teach you why a force against light pressure can be generated. In both cases you will need some basic knowledge on ray optics. You may refer either to Appendix A1 and A2 or to the "crash course" in Box 28.

### Box 28: A crash course in ray optics

In spite of the fact that light is a wave, its interaction with sufficiently large objects can be described by the propagation of rays. A ray, theoretically, is a thin beam of light and may be represented on paper by a straight line. In contrast, a real beam has a diameter of at least the wavelength and has to be represented by a large number of rays. The optical behavior of a beam can often be characterized by a small number of selected rays.

The refractive index of a medium quantifies how much a ray of light changes its direction when it enters the medium from, for example, the vacuum (or from air as a good ap-proximation).

When a ray comes from a medium with a small refractive index into a medium with a high refractive index, it changes its direction towards the surface normal. The latter is the line perpendicular to the tangent in the point of impact of the ray.

The surface normal through a point of a sphere is the radius, i.e. the surface normal is de-fined by the point of impact and the center of the sphere.

By a convex spherical surface of glass, rays in a beam of parallel light can only be refracted in such a way that the whole beam is focused. A spherical surface always acts as a col-lecting lens.

Rays in a *highly focused* beam of light can be refracted in such a way as to *defocus* the whole beam.

## 2.5.2 Why are particles pushed towards the optical axis?

A simple explanation uses the fact that most biological objects are partially transparent for light and have an index of refraction larger than the buffer solution in which they are suspended. In most cases they have a curved surface. For simplicity one can assume a spherical surface. Thus they resemble lenses in which light is diffracted, i.e. upon entering the sphere the path of light changes its direction towards the surface normal. Upon change of direction a ray of light transfers momentum to the environment. Fig. 17 (modified from Ashkin and Dziedzik, 1989) illustrates this and shows how the different forces add up to a resulting force directed towards the optical axis. Note one important detail: so far no assumption has been made that the light is focused. The effect works equally well with focused and with completely parallel light.

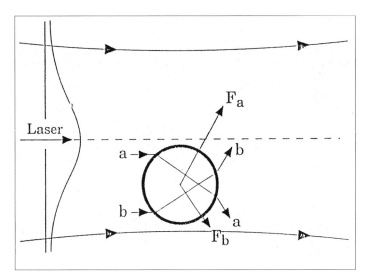

**Fig. 17:** *Stabilizing a dielectric sphere on the optical axis. Light is refracted for example by a cell with higher refractive index than the solvent. The change in direction causes momentum transfer from light onto the cell. In the ray with the label «a» the light gains momentum directed away from the center of the beam (the optical axis). Since total momentum of the system has to be conserved, the cell gains momentum towards the beam center. In contrast, ray «b» causes a momentum driving the cell out of the beam. If the laser beam were homogeneous, all transversal forces would ultimatelly cancel each other and only light pressure would be observed. Since the light intensity in beam «b» is smaller than in beam «a», a total momentum directed to the center of the laser beam results.*

## 2.5.3 Why are particles pulled against the light pressure force?

The previous considerations do not explain why a particle can be pulled into the focus even against the direction of light propagation. You know that light pressure tends to push the particle away. The magnitude of light pressure depends on the intensity of the laser beam. In contrast, the gradient force depends on the change of the electric field in three dimensional space. For simplicity, we assume here, that the electric field E has a gradient only along the z-axis, i.e. along the direction of light propagation. Then

$$F_{gradient} = D \cdot dE/dz \quad (33)$$

where D is the dipole moment of the object to be trapped. Since light pressure can be made large, one has to take care that dE/dz is also large. It is virtually impossible to achieve this with unfocused light and it is most efficient when the trapping laser is focused with the highest possible numerical aperture, ideally NA=1.3 or 1.4.

Again, ray optics gives a surprisingly simple explanation of the counterintuitive process: Fig. 18 from Ashkin and Dziedzik, 1989 shows how the stabilizing forces can work. For details see the figure caption.

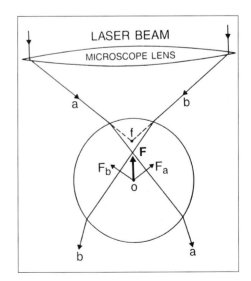

**Fig. 18:** *The laser beam is characterized by the rays «a» and «b.» Its focus «f» is closer to the light source than the center of the sphere, «O». Since the index of refraction of the sphere is larger than that of the environment, ray «a» is refracted towards the surface normal, i.e. the dotted line through O and A. Similarly as in Fig. 17 this causes a change in momentum. The sphere reacts with a force Fa in the opposite direction (only Fa is drawn). The situation for ray «b» is similar. The resulting force F can be found by adding Fa and Fb as shown (since forces behave as vectors). F is directed towards the light source. As long as F is larger than the light pressure, the sphere will be pulled back towards the light source. With a less pronounced focusing, F will only be small and may never cancel light pressure. Therefore, a sharp focusing (with high numerical aperture) is mandatory.*

## 2.5.4 Quantitative influence of objective illumination and of refractive index

Not only should focusing be performed with a high NA objective. The objective should also be optimally illuminated by the trapping laser. One might think that the best trapping effect is achieved when the laser just barely fills the aperture of the objective on the side of the light sources (i.e. on the opposite side from the object). Often this aperture is called the exit pupil. Such an illumination is good but, in fact, not optimal. When the beam of the trapping laser is expanded to infinity, the pupil is illuminated homogeneously and this causes the highest trapping effect. When the beam is expanded to fit almost exactly the diameter of the pupil, the trapping effect is 87% of the optimum, but much less total laser power will be required. Only when the exit pupil is underilluminated, does the trapping strength rapidly decrease.

A second important quantity is the influence of the ratio $n/n_1$ (the effective index of refraction) on the gradient force. For a polystyrene sphere (n=1.6) in water ($n_1$=1.33) this value is 1.2. Box 29 shows the effect of $n/n_1$ on F, which is arbitrarily assumed to be 100% at a refractive index ratio of $n/n_1$=1.2.

**Box 29: Magnitude of the stabilizing force component "F" for different refractive index ratios $n/n_1$. The value at $n/n_1$=1.2 (polystyrene sphere in water) is arbitrarily set at 100%: Data from Ashkin (1992).**

| $n/n_1$ | F |
|---------|--------|
| 1.05 | 61.9 % |
| 1.1 | 90.2 % |
| 1.2 | 100 % |
| 1.3 | 112.5 % |
| 1.4 | 110.2 % |
| 1.6 | 92.5 % |
| 1.8 | 66.7 % |
| 2.0 | 37.9 % |

A good performance of the laser trap can be achieved approximately over the range $n/n_1$=1.1 to 1.6, in which most biological samples in physiological solutions are found. Here it has to be mentioned that laser beams can have cross sections other than the here assumed Gaussian beam profile; for example, ring-like or doughnut cross sections. At high refractive index ratios, cross sections such as these are more suitable. For details see Ashkin (1992).

 Several general conclusions can be drawn:

1. The axial trapping force depends on the distance of the microsphere from the coverglass.
2. In the ray optics regime (5 μm and above) the axial force is relatively insensitive to sphere radius, but changes dramatically when the diameter approaches the wavelength.
3. The transversal force depends slightly on the polarization of the laser.
4. The transversal forces depend significantly on the sphere size.
5. Theoretical predicitions are good in the range for which they are made. In the transition range they are poor.

## Summary and outlook

 Unlike light pressure, gradient forces allow the pulling of dielectric particles against the direction of light propagation. In order to achieve significant effects it is, however, necessary to focus a laser with high numerical aperture. Then one has three-dimensional control over microscopic objects.

## Selected references

A. Ashkin and J.M. Dziedzic (1989) Optical trapping and manipulation of single living cells using infrared laser beams. Ber. Bunsenges. Phys. Chem. 93, 254–258.

Ashkin (1992) Forces of a single-beam gradient laser trap on a dielectric sphere in the ray optics regime. Biophys. J. 61, 569–582.

W.H. Wright, G.J. Sonek and M.W. Berns (1994) Parametric study of the forces on microspheres held by optical tweezers. Applied Optics 33, 1735–1748.

# 2.6 Unprecedented accuracy and precision: Nanometers and piconewtons

With the theory and the techniques reported in the previous chapters it is possible to exert and measure forces within an accuracy of, say, 30%. While even this is quite useful for most experiments in biotechnology and biomedicine, optical tweezers can be much more precise: they can be used as picotensiometers: positions can be measured with nanometer reproducibility and forces with piconewton accuracy. This is several hundred times more accurate than the resolution of a light micro-cope (although reproducibility is not really "resolution" in the strict sense) and it is several 1000 times finer than the force of a single covalent chemical bond! It may be not too surprising that in order to achieve such unprecedented accuracy, a bit of sophisticated calibration is required.

Calibration of force measurement means finding a correlation between laser power and the forces acting in the microscopic world. Basically four different calibration strategies have been developed. Two of them (the escape force and the trap stiffness method) measure how the optical trap counteracts viscous forces. The two others (the corner frequency and the minimal information method) use thermal fluctuations for calibration. An excellent overview on calibration methods is available from Svoboda and Block (1994).

## 2.6.1 The escape force method for calibrating optical tweezers

The conceptually and experimentally simplest approach to calibrate optical tweezers is the escape force method. At a preset laser power, the object is held in a flow of liquid of increasing velocity until the object escapes. The object's velocity immediately after escape is assumed to be equal to the velocity of the liquid. The Stoke's law (Box 30) then allows one to correlate the preset laser power to the escape force. Repeating this experiment for other laser powers gives a calibration curve "force versus laser power", which will be valid for other experiments as long as shape, refractive index and laser geometry are similar to that in the calibration experiment.

One way to perform this experiment is to move a motor or piezo-driven x-y stage for the microscope and to hold a microbead with the optical tweezers, i.e. the complete environment is moved and the relative velocity is determined by the velocity of the stage.

In spite of its simplicity, the escape force method has a disadvantage: Spherical aberration due to refractive index mismatch at the glass/solution interface or changes in the effective viscosity close to the surface (see Box 31, reproduced from Svoboda and Block, 1994) may cause errors, particularly when the trap is calibrated several micrometers inside the solution, while the force measurement is carried out directly on the glass surface.

**Box 30: Viscosity and optical tweezers : the Stokes law and Reynolds number**

Any flow of liquid exerts a viscous drag on microscopic objects such as a microsphere. The force can be calculated by the "Stokes law":

$$F = 6\pi \cdot \eta \cdot a \cdot v$$

where $\pi = 3.14$, $\eta$ is the viscosity (for water h=0.001025 $N \cdot sec \cdot m^{-2}$), a is the radius of the sphere, and v is the velicity of the liquid. For example, for a microsphere with 1 μm radius in a flow of water with the velocity of 10 μm/s

$$F = 6\pi \cdot \eta_{water\ at\ 20\ °C} \cdot radius\ of\ sphere \cdot velocity\ water$$

$$F = 18.85 \cdot 0.001025\ Nsec/m^2 \cdot 1\ \mu m \cdot 10\ \mu m/sec$$

$$F = 0.193\ pN.$$

With a liquid such as glycerin ($\eta=1.528$ $N \cdot sec \cdot m^{-2}$) the result is F=288 pN.
The Stokes law looses validity when turbulences occur. This is the case when the dimensionless number

$$Re = v \cdot a \cdot \rho / \eta$$

becomes larger than approx. 1200. Re stands for Reynolds number and $\rho$ is the density of the solvent. The other quantities have been defined above.
Typical objects in optical trapping have a radius "a" in the micrometer regime and a density in the range of that of water, 1 $g/cm^3$. If such an object is in a flow of water with a velocity of 10 $\mu ms^{-1}$, the Reynolds number can be calculated as

$$Re = 10\ \mu m \cdot sec^{-1} \cdot 1\ \mu m \cdot 1\ g \cdot cm^{-3} / 0.001025\ N \cdot sec \cdot m^{-2}.$$

Using the following conversions of dimension

$$1 \text{ N·sec·m}^{-2} = 1 \text{ kg·m}^{-1}\text{·sec}^{-1},$$

$$1 \text{ g·cm}^{-3} = 1000 \text{ kg/m}^{-3}$$

$$1 \text{ mm}^2 = 10^{-12} \text{ m}^2$$

one obtains

$$\text{Re} = 10^{-8} \text{ kg·m·sec}^{-1}/0.001025 \text{ kg·m·sec}^{-1} = 10^{-5}.$$

This is far from any turbulence. When glycerin with more than a 1000-fold higher viscosity is used, the Reynolds number becomes even smaller.

## 2.6.2 The stiffness method

The trap stiffness method uses the fact that optical tweezers at a second look are not really rigid. The arms of the tweezers are "soft". Thus, a mechanical analogue to describe optical tweezers is an object (for example, a microbead) connected via an elastic spring to a fixed point in the trap center. When the bead is exactly in the equilibrium point of the spring, no force is acting (or more precisely: all forces are in balance). When the bead moves slightly out of the laser beam center, a force tends to pull it back. At least at small distances, the force F increases linearly with elongation x, or

$$F = \alpha \cdot x \quad (34)$$

where the proportionality constant a is called the "stiffness".

For a stiff spring (i.e. for large a) a larger force is required to move the bead by a given distance x than for springs with low stiffness. In principle, the stiffness may be measured by statically pulling the bead by a certain distance and measuring the force required to achieve that elongation. This procedure is not very practical for optical tweezers, since the distances are often only nanometers. The "pendulum" approach is simpler: The bead is stimulated externally to oscillate – it behaves as a "harmonic oscillator" (pendulum). Instead of applying a periodic force one can also periodically modify the power of the trapping laser (Wang, 1997). Locally this has the same effect: the bead begins to oscillate and its frequency reflects the stiffness. Due to the stiffness of the springs the motion of the pendulum lags behind excitation. The temporal delay (the phase shift) is a measure for the stiffness (for details see Box 32). A variant of this is to displace the bead rapidly and to measure the delay with which it follows the displacing movement (Simmons et al., 1996).

Once the stiffness of the trap as a function of laser power is known, the force acting on an object held by the tweezers can be calculated after measuring its distance x from the trap center and calculating F according to Equation 34. However, extreme accuracy is required for the x measurement. Section 2.6.5 reports on two approaches to achieve such accuracies.

**Box 31: A source for calibration errors: Drag on a sphere near a planar surface (Faxen's law)**

| (h/a) | Drag relative to drag at h = ∞ | (h/a) | Drag relative to drag at h = ∞ |
|-------|--------------------------------|-------|--------------------------------|
| 1.01  | 2.97 | 3 | 1.23 |
| 1.10  | 2.36 | 4 | 1.16 |
| 1.25  | 1.92 | 5 | 1.10 |
| 1.50  | 1.62 | 10 | 1.06 |
| 1.75  | 1.47 | 50 | 1.01 |
| 2 1.39 | ∞ | | 1.00 |

h = distance of sphere's center above surface; a = sphere radius; at h = ∞ the force can be calculated by the Stokes law (Box 30).

**Box 32: Stiffness calibration by periodic external forces**

Equation 34 disregards the fact that during the calibration process the bead moves at a velocity dx/dt in a liquid with a viscosity $\eta$. Therefore, equation 34 has to be modified

$$F = a \cdot x + 6\pi \cdot \rho \cdot \eta \cdot dx/dt.$$

This equation is only valid for low Reynold numbers, but in Box 29 we have seen that this condition is met in practically all applications of optical tweezers.

Let us assume that the bead is induced to oscillate by a sinus-like periodic stimulus with the frequency f and the amplitude A. Such a motion causes a time-dependent force which in complex number representation is

$$F(t) = 2\pi \cdot i \cdot f \cdot \eta \cdot A \cdot \exp(-2\pi \cdot i \cdot f \cdot t)$$

where i is the imaginary number, $\sqrt{-1}$. Readers not aquainted with this type of mathematical calculus may just delete the i and replace the exponential function exp by a sinus in order to imagine what physically is going on. Combining the two equations above in this box gives a differential equation with the following solution:

$$x(t) = \{A \cdot f / \sqrt{f_o^2 + f^2}\} \cdot \exp[(i \cdot (2\pi \cdot f \cdot t - \delta)].$$

x(t) is the position of the bead in the tweezers at a time t, A is the amplitude of this motion. F is the vibration frequency and $f_o$ is a value at which periodic motion breaks down and which can be measured by varying the excitation frequencies. One can see that the exponential terms in the equations for F(t) and for x(t) look similar, except that the latter has an additional term $\delta$. Physically this means that the bead performs the same type of motion as the object stage but lags behind it. It is this phase shift that facilitates avoiding difficult equations to calibrate optical tweezers. Fortunately it turns out that

$$\delta = -\tan^{-1}(f_o/f).$$

The phase shift $\delta$ can be easily calculated. Then, all figures are known, F(t) and x(t) can be calculated from the equations in this box and subsequently $\alpha$ can be obtained via Equation 34.

### 2.6.3 Calibration by thermal motion: The corner frequency method

In both calibration strategies described so far, the motion of the bead was induced by applying an external force. Alternatively, thermal motion can be exploited (see, for example, Florin et al., 1998). One of these approaches is the "corner frequency" method. Basically, it uses the fact that microscopic particles undergo slight fluctuations in position. In an ensemble of many particles, individual ones fluctuate with different oscillation frequencies. If one measures the amplitude of these oscillations as a function of frequency one obtains a simple curve, as long as the particle moves in a harmonic potential, i.e. as long as the forces are related to elongations via Equation 34. One form parameter of this curve is a quantity called "corner frequency", which is related to the stiffness. However, as in the two calibration strategies above, one needs knowledge of local viscosities and needs to assume that Equation 34 holds exactly, i.e. that the potential is harmonic. For details, see Box 33.

## 2.6.4 Calibration by thermal motion: The minimal information method

Knowledge of the local viscosity is not required in the minimal information approach. This method uses the fact that, under the influence of thermal motion, the elongation x of a microbead is statistically distributed according to the Boltzmann law. The specific form of the Boltzmann distribution contains the stiffness. Experimentally, one takes, say, 1000 snapshots of the position of the microbead in the laser trap and determines how often it is found at a certain distance x from the trap center. From this, a probability distribution p(x) can be plotted and the stiffness can be calculated as shown in Box 34.

**Box 33: Stiffness calibration via the corner frequency**

For harmonically bound particles the stiffness can be derived from the corner frequency of the power spectrum. The power spectrum for a harmonically bound particle can be described by a Lorentzian function

$$A^2_{th} = A^2_o/(1+(w/w_o)^2)$$

where $w_o$ is the corner frequency.

The corner frequency itself depends on the stiffness of the trapping potential and on the viscous force according to the Stokes law (Box 31). This results in

$$w_o = \alpha/(6\pi \cdot \eta \cdot r)$$

where a is the stiffness (see Equation 34), h the viscosity and r is the radius of the microbead. Thus, by measuring the power spectral density versus frequency, with known bead radius and known viscosity the stiffness can be determined.

### Box 34: From the Boltzmann distribution to the stiffness

In thermal equilibrium, the probability of an object having a given energy is governed by the Boltzmann distribution which in essence is an inverse exponential law. For example, molecules in higher regions of the Earth's atmosphere have a higher potential energy than those close to the surface. Only few molecules happen to reach these heights. Therefore the atmosphere is thinner (the pressure is lower) than immediately above ground. Indeed one can, at least in principle, determine the Earth's gravitational constant by measuring air pressure as a function of height. In the optical trap the equivalent to the gravitational constant is the stiffness.

The probability p(x) of finding a microbead at position x, where it has the potential energy E(x) is given by the Boltzmann constant:

$$p(x) = C \cdot \exp\left(-E(x)/(k \cdot T)\right)$$

with k = Boltzmann constant and T = Kelvin Temperature. C is a normalization constant defined in a way that the area (the integral) over the whole probability spectrum is 1. This is satisfied automatically when the measured x values of the snapshots (see text of Section 2.6.4) are represented as ratios or as percentage /100. Then C=1.

In a harmonic potential (when Equation 34 is satisfied) E(x) is

$$E(x) = 1/2 \, a \cdot x^2$$

The only unknown in the two equations is a and thus can easily be calculated.

Note that this is a quite general approach. Any other potential E(x) can also be used, provided a correlation between E(x) and x can be established.

## 2.6.5 Split photodiodes and interferometers for nanometer accuracies

The detectors required for these calibration procedures must be very sensitive and exact, since displacements in the nanometer range have to be detected. One possible solution is the split photodiode detector. The photodiode is divided exactly into two equal parts. When a light-emitting object is located exactly in the plane of the split line, both sides of the photodiode receive the same amount of light. Since photodiodes convert detected light into an electrical signal (voltage or current), the difference voltage or current is zero. When the bead is slightly displaced this balance is disturbed and an electric difference signal can be measured. Since such differences can be measured with ppm accuracies, the split photodiode detector is accurate. In practical experiments, detectors are used which are not split into two, but into at least four fields (split-quadrant photodiodes) in order to measure x and y positions. The spatial calibration is comparatively simple. The x-y table of the microscope and thus the microbead is moved with a piezo-positioner. Such a positioner contains a piezocrystal which changes its length when an electric field is applied. Using sufficiently low fields, nanometer motions can be generated.

An alternative is a detector which relies on optical interference. Interferometers are generally the most accurate pieces of equipment to measure position. They are so accurate that the speed of light (from Earth to Moon in approx. 1 sec) can be measured by a table-top-sized equipment (a Michelson interferometer).

For the measurement of bead positions in optical tweezers the interference of two synchronous waves of differently polarized light is exploited. Two such waves can be generated by passing one light wave through a special type of prism which is called "Wollastone prism". It generates two partial light waves which are polarized in opposite ways, i.e. they have orthogonal polarization. The two partial beams are focused onto a bead. They act by themselves as tweezers and thus they can be used simultaneously to trap an object and to measure position. This is a distinct advantage as compared to the split photodiode. After having passed the bead, the two beams are recombined by a second Wollastone prism.

When the bead is exactly in the center of this arrangement, the recombined beam will have a pure circular polarization. When the bead is slightly out of center, a retardation between the two beams results. After recombination the polarization is elliptic rather than circular. The ellipticity is a very accurate measure of bead position.

## Summary and outlook

By calibration, a relationship is established between the output power of the trapping laser and the force which it generates in the microscopic world. Four different calibration methods are available. Three of them require the knowledge about the local viscosity of the medium. Calibrated optical tweezers can measure forces lower than the force exterted by a single hydrogen bond.

For position measurement, split photodiodes and polarization interferometers are available. They allow one to measure the position of, for example, a microbead with a reproducibility of better than one nanometer. Interferometers allow one to measure positions within an optical trap with high reproducibility as well as with high accuracy, since trapping and position measurement use the same partial laser beams.

## Selected literature

E.-L. Florin, A. Pralle, E. H. K. Stelzer, and J. K. H. Hörber (1998) Applied Physics A, 66, 575–578 Photonic force microscope calibration by Thermal noise analysis.

M.D. Wang, H. Yin, R. Landick, J. Gelles and S.M. Block (1997) Stretching DNA with optical tweezers. Bioph. J. 72.3, 1335–1346.

R.M. Simmons, J.F. Finer, S. Chu and J.A. Spudich (1996) Quantitative measurement of forces and displacement using an optical trap. Bioph. J. 70.4, 1813-1822.

K. Svoboda and S.M. Block (1994) Biological applications of optical forces. Ann. Rev. Biophys. Biomol. Struct., 247–285.

Note added in proof:
A further calibration method has been published in 1998:

G. Fuhr, Th. Schnelle, T. Müller, H. Hitzler, S. Monajembashi, K.O. Greulich 1998 Applied Physics A, 67, 385–390 For measurements of optical tweezers in electro-optical cages.

# From the first simple experiments to sophisticated applications of laser microtools

We are there! We now have a complete set of laser microtools: a laser microbeam and optical tweezers. The microbeams can be used to ablate, drill holes, weld, fuse or to cut. The optical tweezers can be used to manipulate and hold objects. In combination, they allow complete micromanipulation by light. We can now start our journey through the world of applications and use the laser microtools in experiments on biology and biomedicine. On our way we will meet with quite complex applications. But let us start with some simple experiments.

## 3.1 Microbeams in developmental biology

Surprisingly, such simple experiments will be possible with the most complex objects of biology – with whole organisms. Developmental biologists want to find out how a fertilized egg finally becomes a complete organism. How does a single, almost featureless cell start to divide, first into a lump of identically looking cells and finally end up being an insect, a fish or a man? For such studies developmental biologists have chosen some particular organisms: the fruit fly *Drosophila* since its genetics is well known. Even its DNA is almost completely sequenced. They use the roundworm *Caenorhabditis elegans*, because the complete organism consists only of a small number of cells and most individual cells are so well known that they have their own names. In the field of plant developmental biology the plantlet "arabidopsis" is one of the model organisms.

The experimental strategy of laser ablation can be likened to the searching for the bug in a motor. If the motor of your car is stuttering and you want to find out which of the cylinders causes the problem, you may sequentially remove the connectors to the sparking plugs. If the stuttering becomes worse, you have introduced an additional problem since it was not the plug causing the original problem. If removing the connector doesn't change anything you have probably located the troublemaker. In short: by deliberately destroying or severing a part of a system you may determine its function – or its malfunction.

In developmental biology the equivalent to removing the connector is the destruction or perturbation of an individual cell or a group of cells in the early embryo. The function of the pertubed cell in the early embryo can be deduced by studying how such treatment affects the organism's later development. Note that in such studies a property of microbeams is used which is not available from other microtools: the possibility to work in the interior of a living organism without opening it.

Microablation relies on the ability of light to be focused in the interior of a transparent object. Many objects are transparent, at least for selected wavelengths. (This may appear strange to you, but remember that even concrete walls are transparent. Think of radio wavelengths the next time you are using your transistor radio inside a building.)

Lasers are not really mandatory as long as spatial accuracies of a few micrometers are sufficient. This is the reason why microablation by light has been used since 1912 (Tschachotin, 1912). The thermal light of a classical microbeam (Strahlenstich) could be focused into a spot of several micrometers in diameter. The nature of the light source and the comparatively large diameter limited the power density but it was sufficient to induce some interesting photobiological effects. The progress from the classical to the laser microbeams occurred gradually. Strictly speaking, development is still continuing since very useful studies are being performed with classical UV microbeams even today (see, for example, Illagan and Forer, 1997).

The first laser available to the scientific community was the ruby laser with its red working wavelength. It provided very low average power but the peak power and its small focus diameter immediately opened a new range of power densities as compared to classical light sources. When the green argon ion laser became available in the late sixties, higher average powers became available. But it took more than another decade until the full range of interactions could be used.

Let us follow for a while the historical path of ablation studies in developmental biology in order to recall the gradual improvement of the microablation technique. We will start with some selected experiments of these early times of laser microtechniques and end with a discussion describing the full potential of effects to be generated at the end of this century.

Box 35 gives an overview on some organisms for which laser ablation has provided information on development.

**Box 35: Organisms whose development has been studied by laser microablation**

Gall midge
House fly
Cricket
Salamander
Chicken
*Drosophila* (the fruit fly)
*Caenorhabditis* (roundworm)
*Arabidopsis*

The first developmental biologists using laser microablation were satisfied with very simple and almost obvious conclusions. For example, in one experiment glands were removed from larvae of the gall midge by a laser microbeam and it was found that the larvae did not develop further into adult midges. The message is obviously that this gland is important for survival even at an early stage of development. Technically, this experiment is certainly at the borderline between classical microbeam and laser microbeam work and would probably also have been possible with classical light. Other experiments required higher spatial accuracy and thus laser light. Many of these experiments have been reviewed extensively in the books and reviews by Michael Berns and his group (Berns and Salet, 1972; Berns, 1974, Berns et al., 1981; Berns et al., 1991; also: Bereiter Hahn, 1972).

### 3.1.1 *Drosophila*: From the embryos to the organism

The fruit fly *Drosophila* is probably the best studied organism in developmental biology for two reasons:

1  The *Drosophila* life cycle is short, i.e. one can perform a large number of developmental experiments within a reasonable time.
2  A large number of mutants is known. For example, when a fruit fly mutant with a defective gene (genotype) shows changes in appearance (phenotype), it is reasonable to assume that the defective gene plays a role in the development of the affected organ or region as the insect matures.

Fertilized eggs of *Drosophila* first develop into larvae and via further stages into the complete insects.

In the late 1970s an often used strategy of *Drosophila* research was the destruction of preselected cells or cell groups in the egg or in other early developmental stages (blastoderm). The damaged eggs were allowed to develop into larvae (first instar larvae) and the phenotypical changes caused by damaging the egg were quantified. The results of such experiments were then presented as a "fate map". Often the damage was induced by micromechanical cautery, pricking or irradiation with a classical UV microbeam. The disadvantage of these techniques was their poor spatial resolution which caused high early mortality. With the UV laser microbeam (257 nm, 20 μm in diameter, 0.7 μJ) it became possible to damage highly defined sites in *Drosophila* eggs. Among a number of different experiments giving many fate map positions, one experiment investigated the positions in an egg which were most critical for development (Lohs-Schardin et al, 1979). Twelve adequate segments of the egg were irradiated; the position of each was described in terms of its distance from the posterior position and in relation to total egg length. The posterior position thus was set at 0% and the anterior position (the future head) at 100%. After irradiation, the percentage of damaged larvae was determined (for details see Box 36).

**Box 36: Damage in *Drosophila* larvae after microbeam irradiation of eggs at different positions (additional positions were studied in the original experiment of Lohs-Schardin, Nüsslein-Volhard and Cremer, 1979)**

| Position in % egg length | % of damaged larvae |
|---|---|
| 15 | 13 |
| 30 | 91 |
| 45 | 71 |
| 60 | 39 |

Regions in the posterior section close to the middle of the egg are obviously more important for overall development than those at 15% or 60% egg length. A more general conclusion of this work, in contradiction to earlier work with coarser instruments, was that no more than 40% of the length of the egg was important for developing a specific phenotype.

While in the experiments described so far some damage was induced and subsequently the embryo was allowed to develop freely, another type of experiment exstirpated a part of the egg called the "mesothoracic imaginal disc," a precursor of the thorax. Subsequently small areas of the disc were damaged and were reimplanted into host larvae. The additional, though partly damaged, mesothoracic disc gave rise to duplications and triplications of thorax elements and gave information on the influence of small cell groups on development.

Altogether, such studies provided a valuable basis for later experiments when gene probes became available, and this finally resulted in the detailed unravelling of *Drosophila*'s developmental genetics and which finally won the Nobel Prize for one of the experimentors, Christine Nüsslein Volhard.

Halfon et al. (1997) used a different strategy: their plan was not to damage a cell in an embryo, but to alter its gene expression. This strategy is based on the knowledge that slight overheating of a cell will cause the expression of specific genes, the heat shock genes. So far, heat shock was only applied with either single cells or whole tissues or organisms. Using a laser microbeam to heat up, selectively, individual cells in a *Drosophila* embryo caused heat shock gene expression only in selected cells. Since such genes are expressed for a prolonged duration, the fate of the heat shocked cells could be followed during the complete development of the embryo.

### 3.1.2 Laser microbeams study the development of the roundworm *Caenorhabditis elegans*

Certainly the most comprehensive laser ablation studies in developmental biology have been performed with the roundworm *Caenorhabditis elegans*. The genome of this organism is fully mapped, i.e. the arrangement of its genes on its genome is completely known. As with the fruit fly *Drosophila, Caenorhabditis elegans* has two easily distinguishable sides – the anterior (front) end has a nose-like structure while at the posterior end a tail can be recognized. An invagination (the vulva) can be recognized under the microscope and "eating" and digestion can be observed. An anus is visible at the posterior end. *C. elegans* consists of such small number of cells that many of them have been given their own names (see Box 37).

One strategy for studying the cell fate is to sever the cell wall between two neighboring cells. The cytoplasm of the two-cells fuse. How the organism continues to grow depends on the developmental stage at which the cells were fused (Schierenberg, 1984). When a two cell embryo (AB with P1, Box 37) is used, cytoplasm streams from AB to P1, indicating that the internal cell pressure in the larger AB cell is slightly higher than in the smaller P1 cell. The fusion product has now the genetic material of two nuclei. Interestingly, this single hybrid cell undergoes a double mitosis and has finally four daughter cells, as would have been the case without fusion. The granddaughter cells, however, are seriously damaged and an adult roundworm does not develop. When in the experiment reported by Schierenberg (1984) the fusion was induced at a later round of cell division, embryos hatched into adult roundworms. However, most of them had severe defects. Nevertheless, a detailed map of cell cycle times after fusion of several pairs of cells could be generated by this first experiment on laser-induced cell fusion

**Box 37: Names of individual cells in the first division round in *C. elegans***

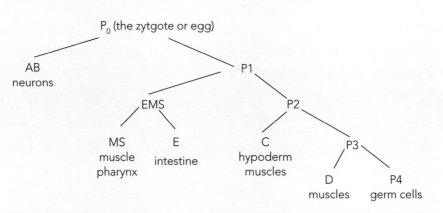

The diagram should be read as follows: The result of the first cell division after fertilization is the AB cell, which is the precursor for all neurons and the P1 cell . The daughters of P1 are EMS and P2, which will have daughters MS, E, C and P3. These will be the precursors for the hypoderm , muscles and germ cells for the next generation. Some tissue types (such as muscle) have more than one precursor. Many neurons also have specific names. These will be given in the text.

### 3.1.3 The nervous system of *Caenorhabditis elegans*

The nerve system of *C. elegans* consists of a very limited number of cells. In spite of that simplicity, it performs tasks as they are known also from higher organisms. Therefore, this nerve system provides a unique opportunity to learn how nerves are connected into neuronal networks and how such a network is used to guide function. Our old strategy, the deletion of individual neurons with a laser microbeam and a test of the neuronal response yields surprisingly detailed information:

The posterior nerve system is the part of the nerve system close to the tail. It consists of only 40 neurons which are interconnected with each other by some 200 synapses. 150 of them are located in the pre-anal ganglion. 12 of 14 pharyngeal neuron classes are collectively required for trapping and transport of bacteria. The class M3 neurons (which are basically motor neurons) in cooperation with 15 sensory neurons trap and sense the bacteria. Other neuron cell classes, ASH, FLP, OLQ feel touch (Hall and Russel, 1991).

A further class of neurons are the chemosensory neurons (named ADF, ASG, AS1 ASE, ASK). The neuron ASE is responsible for sensing (chemotaxis to) cAMP, biotin, $Cl^-$ and $Na^+$. After damaging this neuron by laser ablation, ADF, ASG and AS1 cooperatively take over, but with reduced efficiency. Chemotaxis to a further substance, the amino acid lysine, depends on the neuron combination ASE, ASG, AS1 and ASK. You may notice that ASG and AS1 contribute to the recognition of all mentioned substances, while ASE and ASK are involved in distinguishing between different molecule types (Bergmann and Horwitz, 1991).

### 3.1.4 Other nervous systems

In the neurosensory system of crickets, pioneer fibers appear to be an early manifestation of the neurosensory system. When lesions are induced before pioneer fiber tracts were formed, no neurosensory system developed, while damages induced after their occurrence resulted in only partial damage to the adult nerve system.

Direct inspection of damage on the function of nervous systems is possible when one injects a dye into neurons of an organism. Then this particular neuron can be studied individually. If a dye is chosen which causes photodamage to the neuron when it is irradiated by a laser, one obtains very detailed information of the neuron under investigation.

In a similar approach latex microspheres are injected into individual neural crest cells (in chicken embryos). In healthy cells such microspheres move along the nerve cell. When the neural crest cell is severed by a laser microbeam, the beads move ventrally, i.e. neural crest migration is severely disturbed.

A final type of experiment is just in the early stage of its applications: laser microbeams may complement magnetic resonance studies on mapping brains. With magnetic resonance studies, areas of activity can be visualized and related to a certain task the brain is in the process of performing. So far it is not definitely clear, to what extent the results from magnetic resonance mapping can be generalized, i.e. how much the activity upon a certain task is individually determined. Laser microbeam studies have already been performed, where small groups of cells deep in the brain of house fly larvae were severed. These studies sought to investigate the influence of such cell groups on optomotor flight stabilization. They may be easily repeated with other areas of fly brains which have been previously identified by magnetic resonance imaging as important for performing a given task.

### 3.1.5 Plant root development: Clonal or positional determination of cell fate?

In most animals, organs and extremities are present at birth. No new parts or organs develop. This is not the case in plants. Major parts can regenerate or develop newly. This outgrowth of new parts originates from a special tissue, called meristem. It is located at the base of shoots or roots. Before outgrowth, obviously all cells of the meristem are identical or at least similar. The plant developmental biologists would like to know if the differentiation of single cells during outgrowth of a root hair or of a shoot is pre-programmed in each cell of the meristem (clonal fate) or if it is just determined by position. As with *Caenorhabditis elegans,* laser ablation can significantly contribute to solving this question (van den Bergh, 1995). As a model the root meristem of the plantlet *Arabidopsis thaliana* was used. For this tissue, in contrast to the shoot meristem, it was previously assumed that the cell fate is determined clonally.

In a differentiated root of *Arabidopsis* cells of different size are located close to each other. When, for example, a large cell is deleted by laser ablation, the gap has to be replaced. One can observe this process. Sometimes, the large cell is replaced by daughter cells from the neighborhood. Two outcomes are possible:

1 The gap will be filled by two small cells since the mother cells are programmed to have small cells as daughter (clonal fate)
2 One of the daughters of the small cell will have a large volume since it grows to take up the space where previously a large cell was located (positional fate).

The outcome of the laser experiment was that the daughter of the small cell became large. This did not confirm the previous belief that in *Arabidopsis* root meristem the cells are clonally programmed. The experiment showed, rather, that the cells differentiate according to positional cues.

## Summary and outlook

Conceptually simple experiments entailing the deletion of individual cells in an organism by way of classical and laser microbeams give valuable information on the function of a cell in an early embryo. Particularly the development of the fruit fly *Drosophila* and the roundworm *Caenorhabditis elegans* can be studied by laser microtechniques.

### Selected literature

L. Avery (1993) Motor neuron M3 controls pharyngeal muscle relaxation timing in *C. elegans*. J. Exp. Biol. 175, 283–297.

C. van den Berg, V. Willemsen, W. Hage, P. Weisbeek and B. Scheres (1995) Cell fate in *Arabidopsis* root meristem determined by directional signaling. Nature 378. 6552. 16 and 62.

C.I. Bergmann and H.R. Horwitz (1991) Chemosensory neurons with overlapping functions direct chemotaxis to multiple chemicals in *C. elegans*. Neuron 7, 729–742.

J. Bereiter Hahn (1972) Laser als Mikromanipulator in Biologie und Medizin. Microsc. Acta 71 and 72, 225–241 and 72, 1–33.

M.W.Berns and C. Salet (1972) Laser microbeams for partial cell irradiation. Int.Rev. Cytol 33, 131–154.

M.W. Berns (1974) "Biological microirradiation" Prentice Hall Series on Biological Techniques, Englewood Cliffs, New Jersey.

M.W. Berns, J. Aist, J. Edwards, K. Strahs, J. Girton, P McNeill, J.B. Rattner, M. Kitzes, M. Hammer-Wilson, L.H. Liaw, A. Siemens, M. Koonce, S. Peterson, S. Brenner, J. Burt, R. Walter, P.J. Bryant, D van Dyk, J. Coulombe, T. Cahill and G.S. Berns (1981) Laser microsurgery in cell and developmental biology. Science 213, 505–513.

M.W. Berns, W.H. Wright and R. Wiegand Steubing (1991) Laser microbeam as a tool in cell biology. Int. Rev. Cytol. 129, 1–44.

D.H. Hall and R.L. Russel (1991) The posterior nervous system of the nematode *Caenorhabditis elegans*: Serial reconstruction of identified neurons and complete pattern of synaptic interactions. J. Neurosci. 11, 1–22.

M.S. Halfon, H. Kose, A. Chiba and H. Keshishan (1997) Targeted gene expression without a tissue specific promoter: Creating embryos using laser induced single cell heat shock. Proc. Natl. Acad. Sci. 94, 6255–6260.

A.B. Illagan and A. Forer (1997) Effects of UV microbeam irradiation of kinetochores in crane fly spermatocytes. Cell Motility 36.3, 266–275.

M.Lohs-Schardin, C. Cremer and C. Nüsslein-Volhard (1979) A fate map for the larval epidermis of drosophila melanogaster: Localized cuticle effects following irradiation of the blastoderm with an ultraviolet laser microbeam. Dev. Biol. 73, 239–255.

E. Schierenberg (1984) Altered cell division rates after laser induced cell fusion in nematode embryos. Dev. Biol. 101, 240–245.

S. Tschachotin (1912) Die mikroskopische Srahlenstichmethode, eine Zelloperationsmethode. Biol. Zentralbl. 32, 623–630.

## 3.2 Intermezzo I: Cells and cellular organelles

Section 3.2 from 3.2.1 to 3.2.8 is the first of three sections termed "intermezzo". The purpose of these sections is to give non-biologists a short glimpse at the biology underlying the experiments described in the subsequent chapters. If you are a biologist and therefore familiar with cells, molecular motors, DNA and molecular genetics, you may skip such sections during a first reading of the book. However, some information and data, particularly in the boxes, may prove useful even to the skilled biologist. Thus, at least in a second reading, have a look into the "intermezzo" chapters even if you feel yourself to be familiar with biology.

### 3.2.1 Prokaryotic cells: Bacteria

A cell is the simplest complete living system. Perhaps the simplest cells are mycoplasma. They have linear dimensions of a few hundred nanometers, i.e. they are close to the limits of visibility by a light microscope. The genome (the complete DNA) of *Mycoplasma genitalium* has approximately 500000 bases and 482 genes (see Box 68 in Section 5.3.4).

Other bacteria live with a few thousand genes (approximately 1900 for the bacterium *Haemophilus influenzae*, Box 68). Bacteria, as cells with comparably small genomes need no nucleus, they have their genetic material just within the envelope of their cell membrane. These simple cells without a special nucleus are called the "prokaryotes".

## 3.2.2 Cell membranes

Membranes are layers of long molecules with one hydrophilic (water-soluble) and one hydrophobic end (water insoluble but soluble in oil or fat). Phospholipids are examples. If there are droplets of oil or fat in water, such molecules will bind them with their hydrophobic end and water with the hydrophilic end, i.e. they solubilize the oil droplet in aqueous environment. That is the working principle of soap and washing powders. If such molecules are left alone in water they can do two different things: Either they arrange themselves in a way that their hydrophobic ends are directed into the interior of a hydrophobic core of a sphere and the hydrophilic ends make the surface exposed to water. These structures are called micelles. Or they arrange as pairwise films, (a molecular double layer) with the hydrophobic ends inside the film. Such films can form hollow spheres, filled with solvent. These bubbles are called vesicles. One could think of cells as vesicles filled with a large number of different molecules and molecular assemblies. Cell membranes will be the target of laser microbeams (for microinjection of materials into cells and for cell fusion) and of optical tweezers (in order to measure their flexibility).

## 3.2.3 Eukaryotic cells: Cells with a nucleus

In contrast to prokaryotes, the "eukaryotes" separate their genetic material from the rest of the cell material by enveloping it in a second inner membrane, the nuclear membrane. The material outside the nucleus is the "cytoplasma". The nucleus is, very roughly speaking, the site of DNA maintenance and duplication and of reading the information contained in DNA.

The cytoplasm comprises the major part of the cell outside the nucleus, except in plant cells where essentially empty vacuoles are larger. The cytoplasm, for example, is the site where subcellular organelles such as mitochondria and chloroplasts (see below) are located. There, genetic information, after some intermediate steps, is translated into proteins. This happens in the ribosomes, well-defined molecular complexes composed of ribosomal proteins and ribosomal RNA. The latter has obviously no coding function. It just stabilizes the ribosomes. Some ribosomes are located freely in the cytoplasm; many are bound to the endoplasmatic reticulum, an exvagination of the nuclear membrane. Eukaryotes may be unicellular or multicellular. Some examples for unicellular eukaryotes are listed in Box 38.

**Box 38: Simple unicellular organisms**

*Diatomea*
*Chlamydomonas*
*Dictyostelium*
Yeasts
Protozoa, among them
    Dinoflagellata
    Ciliata (for example *Paramecium* or slipper animalcule)
    *Heliozoa*
    Amoeba (for example the giant amoeba *Reticulomyxa*)

**Box 39: Estimation of the number of cells in the average adult human body**

A crude estimate of the number of cells in the human body can be obtained from calculating weights:

A typical human cell has a linear dimensions of 15 µm, corresponding to a volume of 1800 femtolitres. Assuming that the density of a cell is approximately that of water, this corresponds to 1800 picograms or

$1.8 \cdot 10^{-12}$ kg.

This means that 1 kg consists of $2 \cdot 10^{12}$ cells.

There are no exact data available on how much of the body-weight consists of cells, but 5 kg is probably too low a figure and 50 kg is certainly too high. Thus , as a crude estimate, we obtain

$10^{13}$ to $10^{14}$ cells per human body.

Some of these unicellular eukaryotes will be subject of laser microbeam studies.

*Chlamydomonas* and *Dictyostelium* are close at the borderline to multicellular organisms. For example, *Dictyostelium* cells, in times of shortage of nutrient, organize themselves as a multicellular slime mold.

True multicellular organisms do only exist in their highly organized form. The average adult human body, for example, consists of from $10^{13}$ to $10^{14}$ cells (see Box 39). Cultures of isolated cells from multicellular organisms (cell lines) or single cells directly isolated from the organism are attractive targets for studies using laser microtools.

### 3.2.4 The nucleus of eukaryotic cells

For most of a cell cycle the DNA is decondensed in order to make the DNA accessible for the transcription, replication and repair enzymes of a cell. This state of the cell cycle is called the interphase. Very crudely, the DNA is distributed evenly over the cell nucleus. If one examines this "interphase chromatin" somewhat more closely, one can recognize structure. An interesting question which was posed for almost a century was, whether the metaphase chromosomes are totally intermingled in the interphase nucleus or whether they continue to occupy specific domains. This question has been solved partly by laser microbeam experiments in favor of specific domains. The relevant experiments will be discussed in section 3.3.8.

### 3.2.5 The cytoskeleton and structure-stabilizing intracellular strands

Many cells have quite a rigid shape. They are stabilized by a meshwork of filamentous structures which can be made visible by fluorescently labeled antibodies. Three major types of structures are found:

- actin microfilaments
- microtubules, and
- intermediate filaments.

In many cases these filaments are not only passive structural elements but, in combination with the motor proteins kinesin, dynein or myosin, they serve as elements for intracellular transport.

## 3.2.6 Subcellular structures: Mitochondria and chloroplasts

All organelles have their own envelope. Mitochondria and chloroplasts are interesting since they can be investigated particularly well using laser microtechniques. The mitochondria are those organelles wherein cell respiration takes place. Essentially they are the cell's power stations. They have a diameter of a few micrometers. The number of mitochondria in a cell may vary vastly. Their surface is highly invaginated, i.e. there is a tendency to maximize the mitochondrial surface. The invaginations are called the "cristae". Quite often it is difficult to see them in a living cell and they have to be visualized by way of a mitochondria-specific fluorescence dye.

Plant cells have chloroplasts, in addition to mitochondria. These are the organelles where photosynthesis takes place. Since they contain the green chlorophyll, they are easily visible in most plant cells. The envelope of chloroplasts is quite complex; However, we will not go into this since, for the time being, it is of little relevance for microbeam or optical tweezers studies.

There are other objects inside a cell which have the function of an organelle or are simply looking like organelles. Among them are vesicles transporting a plethora of materials, starch agglomerates and particles which are used by the cell for sensing; for example, for gravity sensing. All these structures are amenable to micromanipulation by light. Here, the specific ability of lasers to work in the interior of an unopened cell is exploited. Their function will be discussed in the context of the experiments performed on them. Fig. 19 shows schematically a cell with nucleus, organelles and a number of structure-preserving macromolecules, with the caveat given in the beginning of this section, that there is no such thing as a "typical cell". In Box 39 an estimate is given on the number of cells in the human body: $10^{13}$ to $10^{14}$.

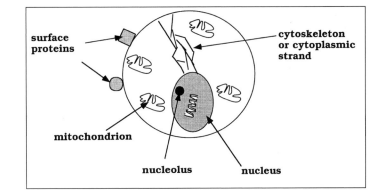

*Fig. 19: Schematic representation of a nucleated cell. Only those elements are shown which are targets of laser microbeams or optical tweezers.*

## 3.2.7 Cell types for work with laser microbeams and optical tweezers

There is no such thing as a "typical cell". In other words, cell shapes and cellular components vary greatly. Bacteria often have a cylindrical shape and have linear dimensions of the order of a micrometer. Protozoan cells have no defined shape – they change their appearance according to environmental requirements.

Cells quite often used in laser microtechniques are blood cells of several different types. Red blood cells (erythrocytes) are the transporters of oxygen in the blood and have a diameter of approximately 6 μm. In birds, the erythrocytes contain a cell nucleus and DNA throughout their lifetime. In mammals, including man, they lose their nucleus during maturation after having synthesized all protein molecules which will be needed throughout their lifetime spanning 60 to 120 days (Box 40).

### Box 40: Lifetimes of different cells

| | |
|---|---|
| Erythrocytes | 120 days |
| Bladder epithel | 66 days |
| Skin epidermis | 19 days |
| Epithel of intestine | 4 days |
| Non-cross-linked nerve cells | 2-3 days |
| Autoreactive T cells | some minutes |
| Cells from eye lens | as old as the organism |

Other non-erythrocyte blood cells also keep their nucleus throughout their lifetime. Among such cells are, for example, macrophages, cells which resorb damaged cells correspondingly marked by antibodies. Another type of blood cell, the eosinophils so-named because they can be stained with the dye eosin, will play some role in microbeam studies. Box 41 gives some basic characteristics of such cells.

Other cells often used are fibroblasts, the major components of skin and other cells of skin like tissues. They have been used especially in older laser microbeam studies because their flat shape allows ready treatment of the interior.

As a particular group of cells the nerve cells (neurons) have to be mentioned. Those neurons which are located in the central nerve system cannot regenerate after birth. They have long spines; the dendrites and particularly the axons in the extreme cases (the axons of the squid nerve cells) can have a length of tens of centimeters. Laser studies will help to study transport processes as well as the networking of such cells.

**Box 41: Cells from blood and the immune system**

**B Lymphocytes**

These are the immune cells which produce antibodies, i.e. the molecules for the humoral (liquid) immune response

**T Lymphocytes**

The cytotoxic T cells recognize and attack cells which are infected with virus. The recognized cells are chemically perforated and killed. A second variant, the T helper cells orchestrate the immune response as a whole. When they are damaged themselves, severe immunodeficiency diseases can occur, such as AIDS.

**NK cells**

The natural killer cells have a similar function as the cytotoxic T lymphocytes, but with a complementary mechanism of recognition. Therefore they often become active when the T cell directed immune response fails, NK cells are not well defined and may finally turn out to represent a whole class of different immune cell types.

Many other cells, particularly prokaryotic cells and some plant cells, have also been studied with laser microbeams and optical tweezers. Since they have often been used only by a single working group, they will be described in the context of the respective experiment.

Box 40 lists the lifetimes of selected cells in an organism.

# 3.3 Laser microbeam studies on unicellular organisms, cells and subcellular structures

Laser microirradiation studies on single cells and their components are performed for several reasons. Irradiation at low intensities gives information on photobiological processes such as UV, visible or IR-induced photodamage to cells. Such studies are, for example, are needed to provide information on the safety of laser microirradiation. The second type of study investigates the function of subcellular structures such as mitochondria, nucleoli and the cell nucleus. Specific structures are irradiated and the change in function of the whole cell is investigated. Altogether the following cells and subcellular structures are investigated by laser microirradiation:

- isolated cells of multicellular organisms,
- unicellular organisms,
- subcellular organelles (mitochondria, nucleoli, nuclei), and
- elements of the cell division machinery.

### 3.3.1 Negative and positive chemotaxis induced by laser ablation

Single cells communicate with neighbors, though not in the same intimate way as cells in an organism or a tissue. In studies of such communication laser microbeams have played a significant role.

The unicellular organism *Euglena* communicates with its environment via chemical signals. When in a group of *Euglena* cells one individual is photodamaged by a laser pulse, the other cells move away from the dead cell. This process is called negative chemotaxis. In contrast, when human blood cells are destroyed by a laser pulse, other cells, particularly macrophages, are attracted and incorporate the dead cell by phagocytosis within seconds. This is positive chemotaxis. Such experiments can also be performed with mechanical microtools, but then a series of blind trials have to performed in order to exclude the possibility that the chemotaxis is induced by the dying cell and not by perturbation through the microtool.

### 3.3.2 Laser microbeam treatment of flagella, cilia and pseudopodia in unicellular organisms

Flagella are structures at the surface of unicellular eukaryotic organisms resembling tails; cilia somewhat look like hairs. They have "motors" at their base and perform a sort of beating motion to propel locomotion. Pseudopodia are sort of foot-like structures which can form and disappear, for example, in amoeba. Any type of severing will affect motility. Therefore, a class of laser microbeam experiments has dealt with such structures. They have been reported in detail by M.W.Berns. As in the previous chapter, only a short overview on the classical experiments will be given here, with some newer experiments reported in more detail.

**Box 42: Unicellular organisms and structures studied with laser microbeam**

| Organism | Structure | Laser used | Wavelength |
|---|---|---|---|
| amoeba | pseudopodia | ruby | 694.3 nm |
| unnamed protozoan | flagella | argon | 514, 488 nm |
| *Oxytricha fallax* | cilia | | |
| *Euglena* | stigma | | |
| *Phragmatopoma* | cilia | | |

In the studies on amoeba it was shown that by irradiation of the frontal zone of pseudopodia the movement of the amoeba was affected. The studies on the flagellate protozoan the function of anterior – posterior axistyle could be evaluated. The *Euglena* studies showed that it is mandatory to irradiate the stigma in order to see a reduction in flagellar motility. The *Oxytrichia* experiments helped to decide a long lasting discussion over two models on the development of ciliary structures. In the *Phragmatopoma* experiments the laser microbeam could be used to alternatively switch on and off the beating of the cilia.

## 3.3.3 Ablation of melanophores in fish

The step from laser micromanipulation of whole cells or cell surfaces to work in the interior was facilitated by the fact that cells contain subcellular structures which are either highly pigmented and thus specifically absorb suitable laser wavelengths or accumulate externally added dyes. For example, cells of some fishes contain granules (melanophores) filled with the dark brown pigment melanin and lend themselves to intracellular micromanipulation. The fish *Pterophyllum scalare* can distribute the melanophores either statistically over specific cells in its skin or concentrate them, thereby changing is colour. Concentration and redistribution is a highly dynamic process with time constants of tens of seconds. Irradiation with light shifts the equilibrium towards concentration. Classical microbeams could not transmit sufficient energy in sufficiently short time to study the dynamics. Thus, Egner and Bereiter-Hahn (1970) used a Ruby laser microbeam (694.3 nm, red) to affect the dynamics. They could show that the cell centre is the organizing centre of the dynamics and thus of the change in colour of the fish. In a related experiment using a frequency-doubled NdYAG laser Rodionov et al. (1987) investigated the fine structure of this concentration change and found that it is obviously directed by ring-shaped fragments of the melanophores.

### 3.3.4 Ablation of mitochondria to study heart function

Mitochondria, the power stations of cells, have ample influence on function. Microbeam studies on mitochondria are quite often at the borderline between photobiology and true ablation studies. Also, since mitochondria are sufficiently large, focusing to a diametre of a few µm is sufficient to induce lesions. Here we have a further example for gradually crossing the borderline from classical to laser microbeams. Work on ablation of mitochondria by light started before lasers were available and only gradually was classical light replaced by laser light.

The majority of the experiments has been performed on cardiomyocytes, i.e. on cells of the heart muscle. The rationale here is to find out what role the mitochondria in these cells play in the organized beating which finally leads to life-supporting beats of a whole heart. Almost all studies investigate influences of light of different quality and intensity on the beating frequency of rat myocardial (heart muscle) cells. By microirradiation such changes of the beating rate can be induced. In one of such studies only a few mitochondria in a living cell were irradiated, but electron microscopic studies revealed that all mitochondria in that cell underwent a cooperative structural change. The interpretation of these results was that all mitochondria in this cell are interconnected. Obviously a concerted action can release calcium stored by mitochondria which may subsequently be used to generate intracellular calcium waves and finally organize the cooperative beating not only of a single cell but of all cardiomyocytes of a heart. Most non-light studies have investigated the beating of groups of cells, since individual cells beat at different frequencies, depending on, for example, the temperature of preparation. When two or more cells come into contact with each other, they coordinate their beating rate. Such studies are interesting when the function of a whole heart is investigated.

These ablation studies were preceded by photochemical and photobiological experiments using an argon ion laser (Rounds et al. 1968). Subsequently, Salet (1970) and Salet et al. (1972) reported a 500-fold concentration of Janus Green in mitochondria and quantified, by comparison with similar effects in model solution of stained albumin the thermal effects induced by a ruby laser (694.3 nm). With a pulsed (Q-switched) and frequency-doubled NdYAG laser (532 nm, $10^8$ W/cm$^2$, pulse duration 30 ns) a somewhat surprising result was seen (Salet et al., 1972). When the cells were stained with the mitochondria specific dye Janus Green, the mitochondria co-agulated and the cells' beating contraction ceased. On the contrary, irradiation of un-stained cells accelerated the beating frequency. Results similar to the latter have been obtained with a classical UV non-laser microbeam. A more direct argon ion laser ir-radiation (488 nm and 514.5 nm) allowed to knock out a definite number of mito-chondria in a cell. At these wavelengths, probably the naturally occurring cytochrome absorbs and performs the task which was taken in the previous experiments by the Janus Green. Many cells survive the knockout of at least 10 mitochondria, corre-sponding to 30-50% of all sarcosomes. The beating rate was affected occasionally, but no definite quantitative relationship to irradiation conditions could be established (Berns et al. 1970). In order to get a more detailed information on the mechanism, Kitzes et al. (1977) recorded the electrical action potential of rat cardiomyocytes af-ter irradiation with a pulsed argon ion laser microbeam (50 μs duration). Basically, small groups of cells were allowed to beat synchronously, selective cells were irra-diated and the membrane potential was measured. Such potentials are significantly different when the synchrony is disrupted – then a special time course of the fibrilla-tion potential (spontaneous irregular activity) is measured. The laser experiments re-vealed that only a special subclass of cells, the pacemakers, were affected. Normal cardiomyocytes recovered quickly after end of irradiation.

Finally, an in vitro study on isolated mitochondria, addressing the site of damage, showed that isolated mitochondria, after laser irradiation, suffer a precisely determined change in the structure of the cristae, the invaginations in the surface of their membrane.

### 3.3.5 Nucleoli

Usually, RNA is transcribed into pre-messenger RNA which is spliced into messen-ger RNA and finally translated into protein. Another type of RNA, ribosomal RNA, instead of coding for a protein, acts as structural element of ribosomes, those organelles where translation from messenger RNA into proteins occurs. Obviously, in order to avoid confusing the two types of RNA, nature has decided to synthesize the riboso-mal RNA in a distinct structure within the nucleus, in the nucleolus. It can be well de-tected due to its high optical density. Therefore, nucleoli became quite early targets of laser microbeam studies. In a relatively recent study, nucleoli in the interphase or in the early prophase (see also Box 47 in section 4.1.1) of PTK2 rat kangaroo cells were irradiated by an argon ion laser microbeam. Daughter cells developed smaller structures, micronuclei. Nucleic acids were absent in these structures. The basic message of these studies was that, in addition to the regular nucleolar organizer regions (NORs) there must exist subsidiary NORs which try to organize new nucleoli after disruption of the regular ones (Hu et al., 1989), though obviously not successfully.

### 3.3.6 Actomyosin fibrils and cytoplasmic strands

Actomyosin fibrils and cytoplasmic strands route subcellular particles through the cell. They are responsible for intracellular traffic. Again, the laser microbeam turns out to be a valuable tool in studies on intracellular motility. For example, the microdissection of actomyosin fibrils in the cytoplasma reveals that the fibrils still can contract. Severing of cytoplasmic strands in plant cells (Hahne et al., 1984) causes the cessation of all motion in the cell, not only along the severed strands. However, after a few minutes, intracellular motion is restored.

In protoplasts of rapeseed, such strands totally disintegrate when a few of them are intracellularly cut by the laser microbeam.

A related study in the alga *Pyrocystis noctiluca* gives an impression of the stabilization of cell structure (Leitz et al., 1994). This cell type has intracellular strands providing a type of skeleton for the cell (Fig. 21a). When one strand is cut (Fig. 21b), the cell changes its shape slightly, but continues to reveal all signs of life. For example, intracellular motions are not significantly severed. Fig. 21c and d indicate that the gap in the cut stand increases with the result of changes in the morphology of the whole cell.

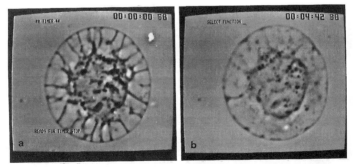

**Fig. 20:** *Microdissection of cytoplasmic strands in rapeseed protoplasts. a: before laser cutting, b: after cutting a few strands. The whole architecture of the cell is affected by cutting approx. 10-15 strands.*

Things change significantly when two or more strands are cut: then the cell loses function. Obviously the number of strands in the skeleton of this cell has been optimized during evolution so that slight damages but not catastrophic events damaging a larger number of strands are survived. This helps the cell to optimize the demand of cell stabilizing materials.

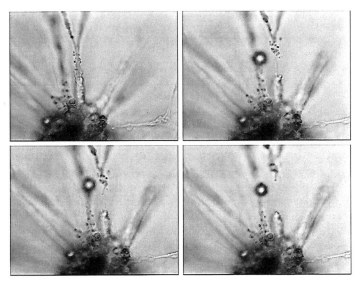

**Fig. 21:** *Cutting intracellular strands in Pyrocystis noctiluca. When only one or two strands are cut, the cell retains its shape. With more cuts, the cell rounds off.*

### 3.3.7 Laser ablation of interphase chromatin in the nucleus

Chromosomes in their compact form exist only during mitosis. During interphase the chromosomes are highly decondensed and not directly visible in the light microscope. This decondensed form of the genetic material is "chromatin" A problem discussed in the literature for more than a century is whether the chromatin of the different chromosomes is totally intermingled or if domains exist in which the decondensed chromosomes still exist as complete entities. The latter model on the internal structure of the interphase nucleus was suggested already a century ago (Rabl, 1885). Laser microbeam studies have given an important answer to this question on the architecture of the mammalian cell nucleus. (Cremer et al., 1982). The detailed experimental strategy is described in Box 43.

**Box 43: Experimental steps to check the Rabl model**

1. Irradiate the nuclei of Chinese hamster cells damaging the chromatin.
2. Allow the cell to repair the damage in the presence of radioactively labelled thymidine. This will be incorporated into the region of previous laser damage.
3. Allow the cell to divide once and to proceed again to the interphase.
4. Check if radioactivity is distributed over the whole nucleus of the daughter cell or if it appears as a clearly defined spot.

When the chromatin is intermingled in the mother cell during laser microbeam irradiation, chromatin of many chromosomes is disrupted. During mitosis it will be distributed over many chromosomes. When the different chromosomes decondense at the transition from late mitosis to the G1 phase it is improbable that all chromatin elements which were close to each other in the mother cell will find each other again in the daughter cell. Therefore, in such a case the radioactivity will be distributed over the whole nucleus. On the other hand, when microirradiated chromatin stems from one single chromosome, radioactivity is concentrated on this chromosome during mitosis and after decondensation will reappear as one single spot.

The laser microbeam experiments showed that the latter is the case and proved the Rabl chromosome territory model. These experiments, performed from 1979 until 1982 clearly helped to resolve a long scientific debate. An additional piece of information came from these experiments: homologous chromosomes are not generally located pairwise in mammalian cells, but in specific tissues; some chromosomes such as chromosome 1 tend to occur in a defined spatial arangement.

Today, with chromosome-specific DNA painting probes available, it is no problem to prove the results of Cremer et al. Nevertheless it was laser microbeam work which yielded the first answers two decades ago.

## Summary and outlook

The property of laser microtools to work at the surface as well as in the interior of living cells allows one to study virtually all subcellular structures: flagella, cilia, mitochondria, nucleoli, actomyosin fibrils and interphase chromatin.

## Selected literature (for reviews see also literature given in Section 3.1)

M.W. Berns, R.S. Olson and D.E. Round (1969) Argon ion laser microirradiation of nucleoli. J. Cell. Biol. 43, 1821–1840.

T. Cremer, C. Cremer, H. Baumann, E-K. Luedtke, K. Sperling V. Teuber and C. Zorn (1982) Rabl's model of the interphase chromosome arrangement tested in Chinese hamster cells by premature chromosome condensation and laser UV microbeam experiments. Hum. Genet. 60, 46–56.

O. Egner and J. Bereiter-Hahn (1970) Laser-Strahlenstichversuche an Fisch Melanophoren. Z. f. wissensch. Mikroskopie und mik. Technik 70, 17–22.

G. Hahne and F. Hofmann (1984) The effect of laser microsurgery on cytoplasmic strands and cytoplasmic streaming in isolated plant protoplasts. Eur. J. Cell biol. 33, 175–179.

Y. Hu, H. Liang and Y. Jiang (1989) Study on mechanism of micronucleoli formation by laser microirradiation. Cell Biophysics 14, 257–263.

M. Kitzes, G. Twiggs and M.W. Berns (1977) Alteration of membrane electrical activity in rat myocardial cells following laser microbeam irradiation. J. Cell. Phsiol. 93, 99–104.

G. Leitz, K.O. Greulich and E.Schnepf (1994) Laser microsurgery and optical trapping in the marine dinophyte *Pyrocystis noctiluca*. Botan. Acta. 107, 90–94.

C. Rabl (1885) Über Zellteilung/On cell division. (in German) Morphologisches Jahrbuch Gegenbaur C, 10, 214-330.

V.I. Rodionov, A.G. Vardayan, V.F. Kamalow and V.I. Gelfand (1987) The movement of melanosomes in melanophore fragments obtained by laser microbeam irradiation. Cell Biol. Int. Rep. 11, 565–571.

D.E. Rounds, R. Olson and F.J ohnson (1968) The effect of the laser on cell respiration. Z. Zellforschung 87, 193–198.

C. Salet (1972) A study of beating frequency of a single myocardial cell. I: Q switched laser microirradiation of mitochondria. Exp. Cell. Res. 73, 360–366.

C. Salet, M. Lutz and F.S. Barnes (1970) Parametres physiques characterisant le dommage thermique selectiv de mitochondires en microirradiation par laser. Photochem. Photobiol. 11, 193–205.

## 3.4 Optical tweezers enter the stage

In the previous sections we have seen the wide range of applicability of the laser microbeam. Optical tweezers came on the stage of biology and biomedicine in 1987. The first reports on trapping living objects were published by Arthur Ashkin's group in 1987. In one paper, published in *Science*, the trapping of viruses and bacteria by an argon ion laser was reported (Ashkin and Dziedcic, 1987). A paper in *Nature* in late 1987 reported that the transition of optical trapping from purely physical applications into a valuable tool for biology was completed by the change from the green argon laser to an infrared NdYAG laser (Ashkin et al., 1997). In these exciting months Todor Buican's group published first results after using lasers to build a micro-cell sorter (Buican et al., 1987). Since these papers represent milestones in the increasing sophistication of this optical trapping technique they will be reported here in some detail.

When it was realized that optical tweezers could be used with living biological cell it was already known from microbeam work that one could work in the interior of unopened objects. However, in microbeam work always some type of severing or destruction was induced in a cell; one always affected viability. With the much more gentle optical tweezers, real vital subcellular micromanipulation became possible.

**Box 44: Optical trapping in the cell interior**

The calculations on energy densities at the cell surface and in the interior performed for microbeams (Box 18 and Section 2.2.4) can be performed equivalently for optical tweezers: For a 1 Watt NdYAG laser the optimal focus has a diameter of 1 mm. Assuming that 10% of the laser power is reaching the focus this corresponds to $10^7$ W/cm$^2$, an intensity at which the first two-photon effects may occur. At the cell surface (5 μm away) only single photon effects are possible and they do usually not cause severe damage in biological membranes.

Among the first experiments with the infrared optical tweezers were also proofs of the possibility of intracellular manipulation (Ashkin et al., 1987). In *Spirogyra*, micron-sized subcellular particles were trapped and moved. Also organelles of protozoa were moved. In a more extended study published in 1989, it was shown that many organelles are tightly bound to their natural position and it is difficult to pull them away (Ashkin and Dziedcic, 1989). This effect was much stronger in *Spirogyra* than in small anions (scallions) where the cytoplasm is obviously less viscous. Also, it was shown that one can interfere with cytoplasmic streaming. In a different experiment subcellular structures were collected and moved in the interior of rapeseed cells (Greulich et al., 1989) and thus prepared for microperforation by a laser microbeam.

Not only subcellular structures can be moved. Obviously also cytoplasma itself can be grasped by the optical tweezers, possibly by trapping structures below the limit of light microscopic visibility. By pulling this material, filamentous structures can be generated which give some idea on the viscous properties of cytoplasmic material (Ashkin and Dziedcic, 1989)

These first experiments were intended to show the potential of optical tweezers in vital subcellular micromanipulation. Quantitative evaluations have not been performed. The experiments described in the next chapter partially repeat these first tests. Now, however, first attempts are made to obtain quantitative information on the interior of a living cell. In this case, the alga *Pyrocystis noctilica* was used as a demonstration object. (Leitz et al., 1994).

### 3.4.1 Optical trapping of viruses and bacteria

In the experiment on trapping viruses, 120 mW of an argon ion laser (working wavelength 514.5 nm, green) were focused by a free microscope objective (not mounted into a microscope stand) with a numerical aperture of 1.25 onto a solution containing the tobacco mosaic viruses (TMV) or *Escherichia coli* bacteria. (Ashkin and Dziedcic, 1987). The trapping events were observed by a photodetector through a microscope from an angle of 90 degrees with respect to the trapping laser, i.e. viruses were detected and analysed by light scattering.

The cylindrical shape of TMV is known, since it was the first virus structure completely determined by X-ray crystallography (see Box 45 on page 124).

The diameter of TMV is much smaller than the wavelength of green light. However, its length is comparable to the wavelength. Thus, TMV is neither a strict Rayleigh particle nor a Mie particle. However, by calibrating the experiment with silica beads of known volume, one can get an approximate estimate of the volume. When the concentration of TMV viruses is small, the photodetector detects light scattering in a statistical way, for example, when a virus enters the volume due to thermal motion. When the trap is switched on, there is a continuous signal registered, which occasionally doubles or triples in intensity, but which will immediately become statistical again when the trap is switched off. It is presumed that one, two or three virus particles are trapped by the 120 mW argon ion laser. This assumption is confirmed by the fact that from the scattering intensity one can calculate a volume of $(45 \text{ nm})^3$, close to the correct volume. Since, for example, the scattering intensity scales with $r^6$ (see Appendix A5) it is very sensitive to volume, one can be confident that indeed single virus particles were trapped. Also, since after several days of virus trapping the scattering per particle does not change, the 120 mW laser obviously cause no major damage in the virus particles.

Since viruses are not really living objects, a final proof for the suitability of optical trapping in biological studies requires vital trapping of real cells, for example, bacteria. The first bacteria ever trapped were contaminations in the virus solutions. During the virus trapping experiments occasionally some strongly scattering particles entered the trapping volume, which turned out to be self-propelled bacteria. In order to observe their motion directly, the equipment was modified. They were now observed through the same high numerical aperture objective which had been used to focus the trapping beam. This was basically the design which is used in modern microbeam traps.

The bacteria could be captured with a laser power of 50 mW and subsequently held in the trap with 5 mW. At this low power the bacteria survived for 10 minutes. A short increase of the laser power to 100 mW, however, damaged the bacteria. The cell content leaked out, similarly as red blood cells leak when they are punctured by a laser microbeam. Analogous experiments with *Escherichia coli* confirmed that, while trapping is possible, laser damage limited the use of the green optical trap. Therefore it was suggested to use other wavelengths to reduce optical damage.

### 3.4.2 The step toward infrared optical tweezers

The final breakthrough came in the same year (Ashkin et al., 1987). A NdYAG laser was used instead of the argon ion laser. Several cell types were studied. Two basic types of experiments were performed: in one type the laser power was determined at which the cells safely survive. Survival was measured by trapping single cells

**Box 45: Size details on tobacco mosaic virus (TMV)**

| | |
|---|---|
| Length | 320 nm |
| Diameter | 20 nm |
| Volume | $(47 \text{ nm})^3$ |

(Index of refraction 1.57)

for several hours and observing cell division. Also, in order to assess the practical use of the optical trap, the speed with which the corresponding cell could be pulled through the solvent without escaping the trap was measured. Box 46 summarizes the results:

**Box 46: Vital optical trapping of different cells**

| Cell type | Power, duration | Vitality test | Max. speed |
|---|---|---|---|
| E. coli | 80 mW, 2.5 h | two divisions | 500 µm/sec |
| Yeast | 80 mW, 5 h | eight cells by budding | 100 µm/sec |
| Red blood cells | 40 mW, minutes | flexibility of membrane | 100 µm/sec |

In the experiments where a single cell was trapped and allowed to divide, the light forces essentially formed a wall-free micro reaction vessel. In the red blood cell experiments the membrane flexibility was determined. Such experiments were repeated as described below (Section 6.4.2). In the second type of experiment, subcellular structures were manipulated in the interior of unopened cells.

## 3.4.3 Single-cell sorters

In the paper described above also a first sort of cell sorting was performed. The E. coli cells were transferred from one vessel into a glass capillary and from there into the volume where they were allowed to divide. At the same time, Buican et al. (1987) suggested a single-cell sorter for routine work. The system consisted of an argon ion laser focused to a diameter of 26 µm by a lens. It was coupled via mirrors into the reaction chamber which was formed so that individual cells could be moved out of a stream of many cells. It had all elements of a modern cell sorter.

However, after the vitality problems with green light had become evident this system did not gain immediate practical importance. Later the argon ion laser was replaced by an infrared laser and the system became available commercially. Even higher spatial accuracy was achieved by Seeger et al. (1991)

The fabrication of cell patterns composed of more than one type of cell using optical tweezers is also possible. Such a cell pattern has the potential to highly facilitate drug testing. With one exposure to a single drug, that drug's effect on the pattern of the whole set of cells can be tested simultaneously. This is of particular interest when cells, differing only slightly from one another (i.e. due to the presence or absence of a specific receptor), are to be tested and it is advantageous to keep their environmental conditions as identical as possible.

A system of five flat chambers on a microscope slide which was produced by silicone polymerization serves as a carrier of the cell pattern. Four of the chambers are coated with material preventing cell adhesion and serve as a reservoir for four different cell types. A fifth chamber is located in the center of the arrangement and is coated with a very adhesive mussel protein /Cell-Tak. It is connected to the four reservoirs by micrometer-sized channels. With the use of optical tweezers cells can be transported from the reservoirs into the central chamber where they, after deposition, firmly adhere to the bottom of the chamber. Virtually any pattern of the four cells can be generated, and be made to contain, if required, different numbers of each cell type. Also, from one population, a subpopulation with a given morphology may be sorted into the central chamber.

The latter then serves as a type of chip which can be tested for interaction with a given substance, for example a drug.

### 3.4.4 Brakes for biological motors: The compliance of bacterial flagella

Cilia and flagella, the cell surface elements which give motility to many cells, have already been studied extensively with laser microbeams. In such studies, the effects of severing or cutting the mechanisms of cell motility were in the center of investigation. Thus it is no surprise that bacterial flagella were among the first targets of optical tweezers studies and publications on them count among the classical work of optical trapping (Block et al., 1989; Block et al., 1991).

The aim of these studies was to investigate the elastic properties of a flagellum. In *E. coli*, the flagellum consists of a long filamentous helical polymer, a motor on the bacteria's surface and another protein having the appearance of an 80-nm-long hook. In a free bacterium, the flagella rotates and thus drives the motion of the whole bacterium.

The mechanoelastic properties of a flagellum can best be studied with bacteria of which the motor is exhausted by starvation or inactive due to a mutation of the genes mutA and mutB which are involved in torque production. The tip of a flagellum can be bound to a glass surface, i.e. the flagellum is then fixed. The bacterium is now fixed to the surface with the flagellum as tether. One end of the approximately cylindrical bacterium can now be turned with the optical tweezers so that the flagellum is drilled either clockwise or counterclockwise. A set of experiments was performed and torsion forces were estimated. The major result was that at small rotations (up to half a revolution) the flagellum behaves like a torsion spring, i.e. the force which has to be applied is proportional to the elongation. However, at larger degrees of rotation, the flagellum stiffens and finally becomes almost rigid.

### 3.4.5 The slipper animalcule survives moving subcellular organelles and the nucleus

A detailed study on the effects of internal cell manipulation on vitality exists for the slipper animalcule *Paramecium* (Aufderheide, 1992). This is an unicellular eukaryotic organism often used as a demonstration object in microscopy. As in the experiments described above, subcellular structures were moved with the optical tweezers. Where the interaction of the laser with such structures was insufficient, microcrystals naturally occurring in these cells were used to push subcellular organelles. Most interestingly the largest subcellular structure, the nucleus could be moved inside the cell over several micrometers. After laser treatment, subsequent cell division was compared with untreated cells. Absolutely no difference in viability was observed, showing that *Paramecium* is not negatively affected by internal cell manipulation.

### 3.4.6 Neural growth cone membranes

Nerve cells are peculiar since, in an adult organism, they generally do not regenerate. However, the spines, the axons and dendrites, can grow, thereby forming new nerve connections. Usually axons do not grow free in solution but on a substrate. In the *in vitro* experiment this is usually just the glass of the microscope slide. Growing axons together with the smaller spines form a cone-like structure. At the tip of the growing axon a dramatic rearrangement of membrane material is required. Upon growth, the leading edge of the plasma membrane must be extended. A shear force due to relative motion on the background resists this growth. The magnitude of these forces, which must be counteracted by the axon's biochemical machinery, depend on the mechanical properties of the membrane at the axon's tip.

These properties can be measured with optical tweezers (Dai and Sheetz, 1995). The principle is that one pulls a sort of filament out of the membrane and measures the force required for this manipulation. However, it is not possible to pull such a tether directly with the tweezers: a latex bead of 0.5 µm diameter has to be coupled to the membrane and then acts as a handle. It has been found earlier that latex beads coated with a special type of antibodies (IgG antibodies) readily bind to neuron tip membranes. When the bound bead is pulled away from the neuron tip, the tether forms and the required force can be measured in the trap previously calibrated by the escape force method (see Section 2.6.1). It is 6.7 pN as compared to 30 pN for red blood cells. Such a result can be immediately understood since a red blood cell, though flexible, needs not grow spines.

The membrane in nerve cells is connected to the intracellular meshwork of structure stabilizing filaments, i.e. to the cytoskeleton. Two models have been suggested: one is that transmembrane glycoproteins bind to actin-binding proteins which finally bind to the actin filaments of the cytoskeleton. An alternative is that proteins such as spectrin are weakly associated with the membrane by noncovalent bonds such as hydrogen bridges. In order to distinguish between both models, the force required for tether formation was measured in the absence and in the presence of cytochalasin B and D or nocodazole, all of which are known to disrupt actin. Since this force is different in the presence and in the absence of these substances, it is concluded that actin plays a role in membrane stabilization, i.e. the first hypothesis is favored by these experiments. However, the quantitative values suggest that the membrane-cytoskeleton contacts are weak, i.e. that probably covalent bond are not involved.

## Summary and outlook

Optical tweezers allow a more delicate treatment of whole cells and subcellular structures than is possible with the laser microbeam. Thus they can be used as single cell sorters as well as a tool to move objects in the interior of cells. The latter function allows one to study, for example, aspects of internal cell architecture.

## Selected literature

A. Ashkin and J.M. Dziedzic (1987) Optical trapping and manipulation of viruses and bacteria. Science 1517–1520.

A. Ashkin, J.M. Dziedzic and T. Yamane (1987) Optical trapping and manipulation of single cells using infrared laser beams. Nature 320,769–771.

A. Ashkin and J.M. Dziedzic (1989) Internal cell manipulation using infrared laser traps. Proc. Natl. Acad. Sci. 7914–7918.

K.J. Aufderheide, Q. Du and E.R. Fry (1992) Directed positioning of nuclei in living Paramecium tetraurelia: Use of the laser optical force trap for developmental biology. Dev. Gen. 13, 235–240.

S.M. Block, D.F. Blair and H.C. Berg (1989) Compliance of bacterial flagella measured with optical tweezers. Nature 338, 514–18.

S.M. Block, D.F. Blair and H.C. Berg (1991) Compliance of bacterial polyhooks measured with optical tweezers. Cytometry 12, 492–96.

T.N. Buican, M.J. Smith, H.A. Crissmann, G.C. Salzmann, C.C. Stewart and J.C. Martin (1987) Automated single cell manipulation and sorting by light trapping. Appl. Opt. 26, 5311–5316.

J. Dai and M.P. Sheetz (1995) Mechanical properties of neuronal growth cone membranes studied by tether formation with laser optical tweezers. Bioph. J. 68. 988–993.

K.O Greulich, U. Bauder, S. Monajembashi, N. Ponelies, S. Seeger and J. Wolfrum (1989) UV laser microbeam and optical tweezers (in German) Labor 2000, 36.

S. Seeger, S. Monajembashi, K.-J. Hutter, G. Futtermann, J. Wolfrum and K.O. Greulich (1991) Application of laser optical tweezers in immunology and molecular genetics. Cytometry 12, 497–504.

# Mitosis, molecular motors and muscles: What laser microtools can teach us

## 4.1 Intermezzo II: Reproduction and motion

How do living things move? What are the forces driving cell division, one of the basic processes of life? These questions captivate many scientists around the world. Nature's tiniest and most efficient motors are the engines of the complex machineries which make biological objects live and move. Laser microbeams and optical tweezers contribute much to our basic understanding of how these processes work.

How does a cell divide? Single cells divide into two copies, grow and divide again. What are the mechanisms and controls which guarantee that the ingredients of the mother cell will be passed on equally to the daughter cells? What are the driving forces? How large are these forces? How is motion generated on the molecular scale - not only the motion which enables cell division but also motion of whole cells, parts of and even complete organisms? How do muscles function? And a seamingly unrelated question: What are the forces involved in the replication of DNA?

Before we can start looking at the laser experiments which have been performed in the context of these fascinating questions we have to learn a little bit about the underlying biology. Therefore, Section 4.1 summarizes some aspects of cell motility. You may skip this section if you are familiar with these aspects of biology. But browsing through these pages might be useful simply for the definitions of some expressions used in the subsequent chapters and in order to learn some quantitative facts about molecular forces.

### 4.1.1 The cell cycle

The cell cycle is the time spanning the period from one cell division to the next. In eukaryotic cells (i.e. in cells with a nucleus) the two major phases are mitosis, i.e. the phase in which chromosomes are visible in the microscope during cell division, and the interphase, in which DNA and the chromosomes are decondensed and can be only visualized through the use of high resolution microscopy or fluorescence techniques. Cell cycle times are very different for different cell types. The interphase is much longer than the metaphase. In a model cell with a cell cycle time of 24 hours, mitosis requires only 1-2 hours, the rest is interphase. Mitosis and sub-phases of the interphase are summarized in Box 47.

**Box 47: The phases and sub-phases in a cell cycle. The complete cell cycle is assumed to take 24 hrs**

| Interphase | G1 Phase (9 h) | Immediately after decondensation of the chromosomes; two sets of DNA are present |
| --- | --- | --- |
| | S Phase (9 h) | Phase of replication of DNA and of production of substances which the specific cells "export to the rest of the organism" |
| | G2 Phase (4 h) | Completing DNA synthesis and preparing for condensation of the chromatin into chromosomes |
| | Mitosis (2h) | Prometaphase (or prophase) Chromosomes become visible under the microscope. Their organization is still unordered. |
| | Metaphase | Chromosomes are arranged in an orderly way and ready to congregate around the mitotic spindle |
| | Anaphase | Chromosomes are separated; in this phase they are particularly elongated |
| | Telophase | Chromosomes are further separated; the borderline between the two daughter cells becomes visible |

During the transition from the interphase to the next metaphase, the nuclear membrane disintegrates into vesicular structures. Concomitantly microtubules, previously distributed in the cytoplasm, arrange themselves so that they have the appearance of a spindle (or rugby ball) shaped basket engulfing the now condensing chromosomes. The nuclear membrane will remain disassembled until telophase. Then it will reassemble into two nuclei immediately before cell division is completed.

The centrioles, short cylindrical subcellular structures, play a central role in this process. Their walls consist of 27 microtubules grouped as 9 microtubule triplets. Looked at from the top, a centriole resembles a waterwheel. Two centrioles are embedded into an amorphous material and form together with the latter the centrosome. As it will turn out the centrosome contains the microtubule organizing centre. At the end of the G2 phase the centrosome is located close to one of the poles of the nucleus.

A second type of subcellular structure, the kinetochore is located in the main constriction of each chromosome. It is the site where the mitotic spindle (see below) attaches to the chromosome.

## 4.1.2 Details of mitosis

Mitosis starts with the duplication of the centrosome. The two centrioles in the centrosome, which are oriented perpendicularly to each other, increase their distance and duplicate so that there are now four centrioles and two centrosomes in the cell.

Microtubules (see below, Section 4.1.4) start to grow in a seamingly unoriented way. During microtubule growth, the two centrosomes are pushed away from each other and end up finally at opposite poles of the cell. The microtubules emanating from one centrosome find the other centrosome and vice versa and the whole system develops the spindle-like shape mentioned above. Some microtubules do not grow in the direction of the other centrosome but in the opposite direction, apparently ending nowhere. Since they have a star-like appearance they are called asters (from the Latin "astra": star). In parallel to this spindle growth the chromosomes have condensed but are located stochastically inside the spindle. Now the pro(meta)phase is complete.

The next phase is the metaphase. It appears that the chromosomes now develop arms to pull themselves into the spindle. Microtubules are now growing from the kinetochores into the empty space. Since each chromatid has its own kinetochore, microtubule growth is observed at two opposing positions. When the microtubules are sufficiently long, they align themselves parallel to the microtubules of the spindle, thereby orienting the chromosomes. Also, they tend to arrange themselves symmetrically in the spindle. The consequence is that all chromosomes gather in the equatorial plane, i.e. in the plane midway between the two poles of the spindle. This assembly is called the metaphase plate. The two kinetochores of one chromosome are always oriented in a way that each of them is oriented towards the other spindle pole. This will guarantee that finally each daughter cell will receive exactly one chromatid of each chromosome. A number of other components enter the stage and the cell is now ready for the third step, the anaphase.

During anaphase the microtubules between the kinetochores of the chromatids and their corresponding pole shorten. Obviously the asters on the other side of the poles form a type of balancing force in this process. This force transmission will also be a subject of laser experiments. The result of anaphase is that the chromatids are pulled towards the two poles of the mitoic spindle and therefore are separated from each other.

In the last phase of mitosis, the telophase, the nuclear membrane reorganizes and a furrow in the middle of the old cell envelope deepens. Finally the membrane closes approximately where originally the metaphase plate was located and the chromosomes decondense. The cell leaves the telophase and enters the G1 phase of the next cell cycle.


## 4.1.3 Details of the interphase

In the G1 phase the DNA is decondensed again. If one would force the DNA to condense in this phase, all chromosomes would be found but they would have only one chromatid. Synthesis of new DNA has not yet started. In the model cell cycle above the duration for the G1 phase has been given as 9 hours. This is correct for cells with a cycle time of approximately one day. The G1 phase may, however, be much longer: days up to years. It is the duration of G1 which finally determines the length of the cell cycle. In contrast, the other phases, S, G2 and mitosis are quite similar for most cell types. The biochemical events of G1 are not well known. The cell is preparing for the major event of the cell cycle: replication. By addition of inhibitors of protein synthesis or by several other measures one can keep a cell artificially in the G1 phase. However, after the cells have come to a specific point in the cycle, the restriction point, the cell will proceed towards mitosis (except, of course, when it is lethally intoxicated). For specific cell types a certain percentage of cells will never leave G1. They are the said to be in G0.

After several hours DNA replication starts at many spots in the interphase nucleus. The starting point are the origins of replication (ORI) which are located probably at distances of 20-40 kilobases on the DNA. Thus, in a human cell one can expect some hundred thousand ORIs. Certain groups of genes are replicated at the beginning of the S phase (early replicating genes); others are late replicating genes. The replication machinery has to be careful not to use a single ORI twice since this leads to gene replication. Excessive gene replication may lead to cancer. Occasionally, such a replication will give the organism a selective advantage (for example, the replication of a gene protecting against environmental hazard) and will be evolutionarily fixed.

For almost a century it has been debated whether the DNA in the S-phase is totally disordered or whether chromosomal territories are still preserved to some extent. We have already seen in Section 3.3.7 that laser microbeam studies have given a conclusive answer to this question. The centrioles, which had an important role during mitosis, are also organizing the microtubules in the interphase.

After DNA replication has been completed the cell enters the G2 phase. As in the G1 phase the cell appears to be quiet. There are indications that a number of proteins and other soluble substances are synthesized only now and that they induce chromosome condensation. This assumption is supported by the fact that, by fusing a late G2 phase cell with a cell of earlier interphase, chromosomes start to condense prematurely. The end of G2 is defined as the moment where, under the microscope, the first condensed chromosomes become visible. The cell now enters the prophase (or, synonymously, prometaphase) of the next mitosis.

## 4.1.4 Microtubules

The microtubules are a driving force behind mitosis. They are polymeric structures made from different isoforms of tubulin monomers: $\alpha$, $\beta$ and $\gamma$ tubulin. They can grow and shrink by polymerization and depolymerization. This growth is partially directional: the plus end is fast-growing, the minus end is slow-growing, so that a net growth goes towards the plus end. In the interphase of the cell cycle, the microtubules are anchored to the centrioles, now elements of the microtubule organizing center (MTOC). Very recently it has been discovered that a central part of the MTOCs is a ring-like polymer made from $\gamma$ tubulin.

**Box 48: Functions of microtubules**

1. Maintain cell shape. In this function the microtubules are part of the network of filamentous molecules, complemented by actin bundles and intermediate filaments,
   which stabilizes the structure of cells.
2. Guide transport of subcellular structures. In this function the microtubules provide a
   type of rail system for intracellular transport. Although they serve in this function in
   many cell types, they are best investigated in nerve cells where material transport can
   cover centimeters- to meter-long distances (for example in the axons of squid nerve
   cells).
3. Separate chromosomes during cell division (as part of the mitotic spindle).

Microtubules are ubiquitous components of cytoskeletons and have, beyond driving mitosis, a variety of different functions in a cell. The three major ones are listed in Box 48.

In all these functions the microtubules are the object of investigation by laser
microbeam and optical tweezers. Laser micobeams will dissect them to study their
stabilizing function and sever them in several different ways to see the consequences when the mitotic spindle, of which they are a part, is disturbed. In the context of motor proteins microtubules will be interesting since they guide intracellular particle transport.

## 4.1.5 Intracellular traffic, cytoplasmic streaming

As Box 48 notes, microtubules provide the "tracks" for the transport of intracellular structures. Actin molecules provide a second type of "rail system.". In order to
find out which of them is driving a specific transport process, one adds substances
to the cell which disrupt or inhibit one or both transporter molecules. For example,
inhibitors for actin are are cytochalysin B. Active transport (in contrast to passive
diffusion of most small molecules in a cell) is particularly important in the relatively large plant cells and in the long spines of nerve cells. In plant cells quite often a vigorous cytoplasmic streaming is observed which is probably driven by actin.
In nerve cells micotubules and their partner molecules are involved in transport
processes. It will turn out that laser microbeams as well as optical tweezers can give
valuable information on quantitative details of these processes.

## 4.1.6 Molecular motors

The "racks", whether they be microtubules or actin, need partners – the "trains" running on them. These are the motor proteins

- kinesin,
- dynein, and
- myosin.

Kinesin and dynein bind to microtubules, actin to myosin; they produce force by conversion of the chemical energy in ATP or GTP, basically energy-rich variants (triphosphates) of the pyrimidine-nucleotides adenosine and guanosine. There are other sources such as glycogen, but they will not be relevant in this book. The motor proteins bind it, hydrolyze it into ADP and phosphate, release phosphate and subsequently ADP. At the beginning of this sequence of events, part of the motor protein (a type of globular head) is bound to a filamentous partner polymer. During ATP hydrolysis, the head undergoes a conformational change with which it moves the partner filament and generates force. The energy conversion rate can be more than 50%. Thus, learning how such motors work is not only interesting for basic science, medicine or sports. It is also of technical importance. With energy conversion rates of far below 20% in technical motors it is clear that understanding and finally simulating the secret of biological motors could result in an enormous energy saving.

The amount of energy which can be provided from the ATP conversion is known. In order to calculate, on a molecular basis, the motional energy which is generated by this process, two pieces of information are required: how long is the relative shift caused by one stroke of such a motor head and what force is generated? Then one can calculate the energy:

$$energy = force \cdot distance.$$

Most of the information required for the understanding such motors has been derived from bulk experiments. For example, the process generating force in muscles has been studied over the last two decades by measuring forces in isolated muscle fibrils. However, in that case some $10^{11}$ motor molecules are cooperating and it is difficult to quantify cooperative processes as well as steric hindrance. Thus the

## Box 49: Forces

$1 \text{ dyn} = 10^{-5} \text{ Newton}$, $pN = piconewton = 10^{-12} \text{ Newton}$, $kN = kilonewton$

| | |
|---|---|
| Hydrogen bond | 300 pN |
| carbon-carbon bond | 30000 pN |
| | |
| Streptavidin – biotin bond | 250 pN |
| avidin and biotin bond | 160 pN |
| avidin and iminobiotin bond | 85 pN |
| | |
| Protein–protein interaction | |
| with a dissociation constant of $10^{-5}$ | 11-22 pN |
| with a dissociation constant of $10^{-7}$ | 32-1400 pN |
| with a dissociation constant of $10^{-9}$ | 74-3300 pN |
| antigen-antibody interaction | 244 +/- 20 pN |
| | |
| Force to break DNA | 480 pN |
| Elastic structural transition of DNA | 65-70 pN |
| Straightening DNA kinks | 6 pN |
| | |
| Maximum force exerted by the mitotic spindle | 700 pN |
| Motility force of a sperm cell | 40 pN |
| Traction force of a locomoting cell | 45000 pN |
| | |
| Optical tweezers (1064 nm), 1 Watt in object plane | |
| pure light pressure (at some distance from focus) | 5 000 pN |
| against light pressure (close to focus) | 150-500 pN |
| perpendicular to beam propagation | 1 500 pN |
| | |
| Myosin, average force during stroke | 2.1 pN |
| Myosin, peak force during stroke | 5.9 pN |
| | |
| Myosin | 100 kN/m$^2$ |
| DNA | $1.11 \cdot 10^{15}$ kN/m$^2$ |

bulk of experiments may give good rough estimates, but single motor measurements are required to get the final answer on energy conversion and mechanisms.

For example it is still open to discussion as to whether the conversion of one ATP molecule into ADP plus energy results in one single stroke of a motor head or if this energy is distributed over many strokes. In other words, one does yet not know whether the hydrolysis of one ATP molecule is coupled tightly to one mechanical motion (tight coupling) or distributed over several motions (loose coupling). This question is also related to the type of energy conversion: since some motor proteins (dynein and myosin) have two globular heads which can attach to their binding partners (microtubules or actin respectively), a model has been postulated whereby one head is bound while the second head moves along the partner molecule, bypassing the bound counterpart (the "hand-on" model; the question then is whether the presence of two heads is essential. Alternatively, each head might in principle perform the same task, working independently from one another. In Section 4.3 you will learn more on this aspect.

### 4.1.7 Forces generated by single molecules

With such experiments we are approaching the field of single molecule research. Indeed, experimental techniques are now sufficiently sensitive for measuring, for example, forces between individual molecules. One instrument capable of performing such fine measurements is the tip of an atomic force microscope. The other instrument is the optical tweezers. Since such measurements require a delicate calibration procedure it is essential to have a large number of known calibrating forces. Such information is rare in the literature. Therefore, in Box 49 a number of known intermoleculear forces is collected from quite different sources, which are summarized in the subsequent list of selected publications.

### Literature for Box 49

D. Bensimon, A. Simon, V. Croquette and A. Bensimon (1995) Stretching DNA with a receding meniscus: experiments and models. Phys. Rev. Lett. 74, 4754–4757.

H. Berendsen (1996) Biomolecular dynamics comes of age. Science 271, 954–955.

P. Cluzel, A. Lebrun, C. Heller, R. Lavery, J.L. Viovy, D. Chatenay and F. Caron (1996) DNA: An extensible molecule. Science 271, 792–794.

E.L. Florin, V.T. Moy and H.E. Gaub (1994) Adhesion forces between individual ligand – receptor pairs. Science 264, 415–417.

H. Grubmüller, B. Heymann and P. Tavan (1996) Ligand binding: Molecular mechanics calculation of the streptavidin – biotin rupture force. Science 271, 997–999.

P. Hintersdorfer, W. Baumgartner, H.J. Gruber, K. Schilcher and H. Schindler (1996) Detection and localization of individual antigen-antibody recognition events by AFM. Proc. Natl. Acad. Sci. 93.8, 3477–3481.

A. Isijima, H. Kojima, H. Higuchi, Y. Harada, T. Funatsu and T. Yanagida (1995) Multiple- and single molecule analysis of the actomyosin motor by nanometre-piconewton manipulation with a microneedle: Unitary steps and forces. Bioph. J. 70, 383–400.

G. Jannink, B. Duplantier and J.L. Sikorav (1996) Forces on chromosomal DNA during anaphase. Bioph. J. 71,451–465.

S.C. Kuo and D.A. Lauffenberger (1993) Relationship between receptor/ligand binding affinity and adhesion strength. Bioph. J 65, 2191–2200.

## 4.2 What drives cell division? Laser microtools help to find the answer

We have already discussed the use of the microbeams in developmental studies (Section 3.1); a second use is the investigation of the mitotic apparatus. These two examples demonstrate how classical microirradiation is gradually shifting to laser microsurgery. In this field of biology, laser- and classical microbeams coexist until today. The classical microbeams are used by the group of A. Forer (for example, Spurck et al., 1997). When small elements of the mitotic spindle such as centromeres or centrioles are investigated, laser microbeams offer some advantage, but often either type of microbeams is equally well suited. This type of investigation deals primarily with the forces which, during cell division, pull the two sets of chromosomes apart and distribute them equally to the two daughter cells.

## 4.2.1 From the early days to complete micromanipulation by laser light

Michael Berns' group started these investigations in the early 1970s. (Berns et al., 1969 a and b, 1970; Berns and Floyd, 1971; Berns, 1974). In these days lasers could be focused to diameters of a few micrometers.

Combination of laser microbeam and optical tweezers allow complete micromanipulation of structures involved in mitosis. Therefore experiments have been designed where chromosome arms were microdissected with the microbeam and then moved with the tweezers within the spindle. Such experiments were of limited success in PTK cells, since there is a narrow cage of intermediate filaments around the spindle. In lung cells from newt, chromosome segments could be moved over significant distances. (Liang et al., 1994). The reason for this freedom of movement is that here the cage is much wider, with a clear zone existing between spindle and the outer part of the cell.

## 4.2.2 Kinetochores and centrosomes: The secret of symmetric distribution of chromosomes

Obviously the effect of laser irradiation depends on the specific phase of mitosis (Box 47 in Section 4.1). This is confirmed by a detailed study on kinetochore irradiation.

When, in the early phase of chromatid separation (in the prometaphase or in the metaphase) the kinetochore of a selected chromatid of a PtK2 cell is irradiated with a frequency-doubled NdYAG laser, the subsequent mitosis is disturbed (McNeill and Berns, 1981). The complete chromatid pair migrates towards the pole to which otherwise only the non-irradiated chromatid would migrate. Neither chromatids separates until anaphase and even then they are separated only marginally (1–2 µm). Surprisingly, the velocity of poleward migration for the chromatid pair is almost the same as for single chromatid in unirradiated cells. This indicates that the underlying forces are strong and that single kinetochore can move considerably larger masses than just one chromatid.

Each chromatid has one kinetochore and it is reasonable to assume that their pairwise distribution onto the daughter cells guarantees equal distribution of chromsomes to the daughter cells. A laser microbeam study at 532 nm has given important information on the underlying mechanism (Skibbens et al., 1995): When only one kinetochore has contact with the spindle, the chromatid pair migrates almost along a random walk (directional instability). Immediately after the sister kinetochore has also gained contact with the spindle, the motion becomes oriented in way that will finally separate the chromatid pair. However, when the chromosome material between the two kinetochores is weakened by very precise laser microirradiation, the motion again becomes more random. Obviously, tension between the two sister kinetochores regulates directional stability. Only when there is tension, will the chromatids be separated symmetrically.

When the centrosomes are irradiated in early anaphase, there is chromosome movement towards the irradiated pole, but not towards the undamaged pole, stops. The division into the two daughter cells is highly retarded. (Uzbekow et al., 1995).

The latter experiments were performed with a classical UV microbeam and show that this device, for some applications, is as useful as the laser microbeam.

## 4.2.3 Microablation studies on intranuclear metaphase chromosomes

Bern's group investigated cells from lung tissue explants of salamander. (These cells are flat and transparent and one can directly see individual metaphase chromosomes when the cells are in the process of dividing.)

Possible effects of laser irradiation on different phases of cell division were studied at the prophase, metaphase, anaphase and telophase stages. Two basic ideas were behind these experiments. In previous experiments whole cell irradiation was found to block mitosis. Possible reasons for this damage may be photodamage to some critical molecules or damage to microscopically visible elements of the mitotic apparatus.

By deletion of specific chromosomal regions and subsequent analysis of defects in daughter cells a type of positional cloning was attempted, long before corresponding molecular biological techniques were available.

A continuous green argon ion laser (wavelength 514 nm) was used. Since chromosomes do not absorb very well in this wavelength range they had to be stained with acridine orange. This dye was thought not to interfere with the vital processes in the cell. Although the primary binding sites of acridine orange in a cell are the lysosomes (subcellular particles containing lytic material) some binding occurs on the chromosomes. The staining procedure is surprisingly simple. The cell has to be held in culture for 1 to 3 weeks nonetheless. Approximately five minutes before the cells are used, acridine orange is added to the culture medium so that its final concentration is $10^{-5}$ to $10^{-6}$ percent. The cell incorporates the dye and it binds to its target.

One type of study investigated differences between cells kept in culture not longer than 2 weeks and cells which had been cultured for longer periods: When chromosomes were irradiated *in the early phases* of cell division (prophase and metaphase) cell division in the long-term cultured cells stopped. The cell had greatly deteriorated, although it did not die. Severing their chromosomes *after* the metaphase did not result in serious damage to the cell: it continued to divide; daughter cells were formed. In contrast, short-term culture cells were not severely affected by the laser treatment in any of the phases (for a short summary see Box 50).

**Box 50**

|  | Irradiation early mitosis | Irradiation later mitosis |
|---|---|---|
| 3–4-week-culture | severe damage | daughter cells formed |
| 1–2-week-culture | daughter cells formed | daughter cells formed |

These results demonstrated that whole parts of chromosomes can be severed without killing the cell. The lesion diameters on the chromosomes were larger than 0.5 µm, corresponding to 1% of the genome or to some tens of megabases of DNA; this reveals that a cell has considerable potential to compensate for gene losses. The fact that long-term culture makes the cells more sensitive to this type of irradiation indicates that culturing cells reduces this compensation potential.

The laser microbeam has also been used to knock out a specific group of genes: in the chromosomes of salamander lung cells a morphologic marker (a secondary constriction or nucleolar organizer region) can be recognized which is known to contain genes involved in the development of nucleoli. A normal salamander lung cell develops up to three nucleoli. Irradiation of the secondary constriction region in the chromosomes resulted in loss of one or two of these. A later study showed that when the secondary constriction is missed by as little as 0.25 µm an effect on nucleolus formation is no longer observed. Obviously, genes responsible for the formation of nucleoli have been knocked out by laser irradiation. On the other hand, the surviving cells with one nucleolus indicate that the number of nucleoli is not optimized for mere survival, i.e. spare nucleoli are present in salamander lung tissue cells.

In these first studies it was not known which type of molecule in the chromosomes was damaged. The major components of chromosomes are DNA and the histone proteins. A subsequent study managed to sever both these molecule types selectively: In the presence of acridine orange at low laser power the DNA was damaged. Without dye but at increased laser power, it was shown that the major damage occurred to the histones. The photomechanism of histone damage could not be explained, since histones have no specific absorption bands at 488 nm and 514 nm, the working wavelengths of the argon ion laser used in this study. However, the possibility of two-photon effects was discussed since chromatin readily absorbs at the half wavelengths of 244 nm and 257 nm. Thus, this 1971 work may be (one of) the first on two-photon effects on a living object (Berns and Floyd, 1971).

The fact that functions in a genome could be deleted very specifically by precise laser microirradiation promote experiments affecting chromosome distribution during mitosis. It was reasoned that deletion of the kinetochore, that structure in the primary constriction (centromere) of the chromosome from which microtubules grow and contribute in forming the mitotic spindle, might affect the fate of the chromosome. For these studies PTK cells of the rat kangaroo were used. Rat kangaroo has only six pairs of chromosomes. A special cell line, PTK2 has one chromosome in addition. The largest chromosome, number 1, occurs in three copies. Thus 2n=13. It was this chromosome which was irradiated either in parts, totally or in the region where the kinetochore is located. The last type of experiment was particularly interesting. In some cases, chromosome 1 with irradiated kinetochore did not go into anaphase and telophase and was lost. This loss could be observed by a time-lapse video recording and it could clearly be seen that this chromosome left the spindle and was lost to the cytoplasma. Therefore, a cloning assay was developed in view of the possibility to develop cell lines with a modified chromosome number. Of 102 cells irradiated in a preselected area of chromosome 1 nine cells could be cloned into viable populations. Five of them exhibited partial DNA deletion on the long arm of chromosome 1; two cells had an entire chromosome deleted. The overall result showed that deletion of a region up to 1 micrometer in size did not cause chromosome loss. A safe selective deletion of one preselected chromosome was not possible.

## 4.2.4 Micotubule polymerization dynamics and flexibility

Other prominent structures in mitosis are the microtubules. They, in cooperation with motor proteins, power the process of cell division. Thus, knowledge on formation and mechanical properties of microtubules is required for fully understanding the action of the mitotic spindle. Growth was studied with the help of a laser microbeam (Tao et al., 1988), flexibility with optical tweezers (Kurachi et al., 1995, Felgner et al., 1996). (For beam data, see Box 51.)

**Box 51: Data on the laser microbeam and of optical tweezers**

**laser microbeam**
Pulsed NdYAG laser
wavelength             266 nm (fourth harmonic)
Energy per pulse:      100 µJ
pulse duration         10 ns

**Optical tweezers**
Continuous NdYAG laser
wavelength             1064 nm (ground wave)
power                  up to 700 mW

The microtubuli of PTK2 cells in the interphase were ablated in a region 5 µm across, approximately 20 µm from the periphery. Some 20 seconds after laser ablation, the cells were fixed in formaldehyde and incubated with an antibody against tubulins, the building blocks of microtubuli. The anti-tubulin antibody is visualized with the aid of a second, fluorescently labeled antibody. In other words, regrowth into the area of deletion was stopped after 20 seconds and the effect was observed using fluorescence staining. Two models of growth exist: the treadmilling model and the dynamic instability model (GTP cap). For each, a different outcome of the laser ablation experiment is expected (see Box 52).

In most cases, situations 1–3 of Box 52 are observed, i.e. the zone of laser ablation increases with time. Thus, the GTP cap model, as a variant of the dynamic instability model, appears to be correct.

For flexibility studies, optical tweezers have been used to bend individual microtubules. In one type of experiment, a microbead was bound to the micotubule,

### Box 52: Predicting microtubule growth: The GTP cap model versus the treadmilling model

#### The GTP cap model

1. The microtubules would grow back into the zone of laser ablation individually, i.e. the replacement of deleted microtubules would occur microtubule by microtubule.
2. The number of microtubules found in the zone in question would increase gradually with time.
3. In a modified version, the GTP cap model, a decrease in the number of microtubules in the periphery would be expected.

#### The treadmilling model

4. The new plus end generated by laser ablation would add and the minus end would lose tubulin monomers. The length of the microtubules would not change and the ablated zone would remain stationary, or alternatively
5. The new plus end would grow at the cost of losses at the minus end. As in 4, the microtubules would behave synchronously.

which could be used as a handle (Kurachi et al 1995). In a second type of experiment the microtubules were directly bent by the optical tweezers (Felgner et al., 1996). Here, axonemes of *Chlamydomonas* were bound to the surface of a microscope slide. In this alga, axonemes act as growth organizing centers for microtubuli. Thus, the microtubuli could first be grown under controlled conditions and then a quantity called flexural rigidity (EI, measured in units of $10^{-24}$ newtons per square meter) could be studied. Two strategies were employed: In a strategy termed RELAX the microtubules were bent at their tip and the flexural rigidity was determined from the speed at which the microtubule returned into its original state. In a strategy termed WIGGLE the optical tweezers held the middle of the microtubule (between axoneme and tip) and vibrations were induced. The amplitude of these vibrations is a measure for flexural rigidity. Microtubules grown in the antitumor drug taxol showed the least rigidity (EI=1.2 units as average of RELAX and WIGGLE experiments), native microtubuli were somewhat more rigid (4.2 units). In the presence of microtubule-associated proteins the rigidity was much higher (17 units), revealing quantitatively one possible role of these proteins.

# Selected literature

M.W. Berns, R.S. Olson and D.E. Rounds (1969) In vitro production of chromosome lesions with an argon ion laser microbeam. Nature 221, 74–75.

M.W. Berns, D.E. Rounds and R.S. Olson (1969) Effects of laser microirradiation on chromosomes. Exp. Cell. Res. 56, 292-298.

M.W. Berns, Y. Ohnuki, D.E. Rounds and R.S. Olson (1970) Modification of nucleolar expression following laser microirradiation of chromosomes. Exp. Cell. Res. 60, 133–138.

M.W. Berns and A.D. Floyd (1971) Chromosomal microdissection by laser: A cytochemical and functional analysis. Exp. Cell. Res. 67, 305–310.

M.W. Berns (1974) Directed chromosome loss by laser microirradiation. Science, 700–705.

H. Felgner, R. Frank and M. Schliwa (1996) Flexural rigidity of microtubules measured with the use of optical tweezers. J. Cell. Sci. 109, 509–516.

M. Kurachi, M. Hoshi and H. Tashiro (1995) Buckling of a single microtubule by optical trapping forces: direct measurement of microtubule rigidity. Cell Mot.Cytoskel.30, 221–228.

J.H. Liang, W.H. Wright, C.L. Rieder, E.D. Salmon, G. Profeta, J. Andrews, Y. Liu, G.J. Sonek and M.W. Berns (1994) Directed movement of chromosome arms and fragments in mitotic Newt lung cells using optical scissors and optical tweezers. Exp. Cell Res. 213, 308–312.

P. McNeill and M.W. Berns (1981) Chromosome behavior after laser microirradiation of a single kinetochore in Pt Kcells. J. Cell. Biol. 88, 543–553.

R.V. Skibbens, C.L Rieder and E.D. Salmon (1995) Kinetochore motility after severing between sister per cent using laser microsurgery: Evidence that kinetochore directional instability and position is regulated by tension. J. Cell Sci. 108, 2537–2548.

T. Spurck, A. Forer and J. Picket-Heaps (1997) Ultraviolet microbeam irradiations of epithelial and spermatocyte spindles suggest that forces act on the kinetochore fibre and are not generated by its disassembly. Cell Mot. Cytoskel. 36, 136–148.

R.E. Uzbekow, M.S. Votchal and I.A. Vorobjev (1995) Role of the centrosome in mitosis: UV micro-irradiation study. J. Phot. Phot. 29, 163–170.

W. Tao, R.J. Walter and M.W. Berns (1988) Laser transsected microtubules exhibit individuality of regrowth, however most free new ends of microtubules are stable. J. Cell Biol. 107, 1025–1035.

# 4.3 Molecular motors: True nanotechnology

## 4.3.1 Optical tweezers and single motor protein mechanics

The motor proteins kinesin, dynein and myosin consist of an elongated part and one or two globular heads. The latter are temporarily bound to partner molecules. Kinesin and dynein are bound to microtubules, myosin is bound to actin. Upon ATP consumption they undergo conformational transitions. Thereby they change the angle between the tail and the head and thus move the partner molecule. After such a stroke the head is released from the partner, swings back to its original position and binds to a new site on the partner molecule. The process is ready to be repeated.

**Box 53: Several questions are of interest for motility research**

1. What is the distance by which the partner molecule is transported per stroke?
2. In molecules with two heads: Are the heads working independently or do they work "hand in hand" (hand-over model)?
3. What forces are generated?
4. Are the forces different at high and low load?
5. How long does it take to complete a stroke cycle?
6. What is the efficiency of energy conversion of chemical energy into mechanical energy (stroke distance multiplied by force)?

In principle most of these questions can be answered by bulk experiments. For example, the force generated by a muscle filament can be measured macroscopically. The number of myosin molecules involved in this process can be determined and from these results the force per myosin molecule can be calculated. But here comes the first problem: The duty ratio, i.e. the fraction of molecules which are involved in force generation at any given instant, is not known and can only be estimated. Depending on the model used, it can range from 5 up to 90%, leaving an uncertainty factor of almost 20. Therefore it is essential to measure these chemo-mechanical processes on a single molecule basis.

One way to measure single molecule mechanics is to use fine glass microtools, but they have their inherent problems such as adhesion and perturbation of the tiny forces involved. Optical tweezers are a second tool for motility research, so that both techniques can be evaluated against each other. The experiments described in the following will make immediate use of the theoretical background and the empirical calibration methods described in Sections 4.5 to 4.7.

### 4.3.2 Force measurements *in vivo*: Mitochondria transport in the amoeba *Reticulomyxa*

In the giant amoeba *Reticulomyxa* mitochondria are transported along micro-tubules. With electron microscopy one can clearly see that the approximately spherical mitochondria with a diameter of $320\pm70$ nm have a few crossbridges lead-ing towards the microtubules they are bound to. Between one and four of such crossbridges are detectable. It cannot be definitely determined if the motor mole-cule is a kinesin or a dynein, but it is assumed the latter is the case.

In one of the earliest and probably the only completely *in vivo* experiment us-ing a laser trap in motility studies (Ashkin et al., 1989) the escape force method was used for calibration. *In vivo* calibration is particularly difficult since the cell interior cannot be ideally simulated *in vitro*. Mitochondria in water gave an escape force of 5.8 pN per mW laser power. Inside the amoeba the calibration factor turned out to be 4.1 pN/mW but it could not be determined exactly what the reason for this difference was.

For the final experiment a mitochondrion was trapped and then the laser pow-er was reduced until the mitochondrion could escape and continue its movement along the microtubule. Escape forces in multiples of

$$2.6 \text{ pN}$$

were observed.

### 4.3.3 Kinesin

First experiments on kinesin-microtubule interaction were reported in 1989 by Block's group and quantified in detail by 1990.

For kinesin, the force motor domain consists of approximately 350 amino acids. It can act as a one single molecular motor *in vivo*, while for example in muscle some $10^{11}$ actin molecules cooperate to generate muscle contraction. In addition, tech-niques to prepare kinesin-coated microbeads and microtubules on microscope slides are fully developed. They have been used to make their motion visible by light microscopy and for the demonstration of high resolution in video enhanced contrast microscopies.

In a typical experiment kinesin-coated microbeads are located on a glass surface covered with microtubules or bundles of microtubules (axonemes). By a suitable reaction condition during loading of 0.2 μm silica microspheres, beads with a large number of kinesin molecules, but also with only one, could be prepared.

After providing GTP or ATP and after establishing contact between kinesin-coated beads and the microtubules, part of the beads start to move along the microtubules much as a train is moving along tracks. Beads coated with a high kinesin density travel on average 1.4 μm. Beads with single kinesin molecules detach soon. A first explanation for this detachment would be that thermal motion is messing up the experiment. But when, instead of ATP, an ATP analogue (ATP-PPSM) is offered the beads remain in contact. Detachment is obviously a result of the action of kinesin.

Subsequently, an attempt was made to measure the forces by using one of the variations of the escape force methods (Section 2.6) by Kuo and Sheetz (1993). They overcame the problem of early detachment. Investigation of 18 individual kinesin molecules resulted in a force of

$$1.9 \pm 0.4 \text{ pN}.$$

Also they found that, for kinesin, the hand-over model is favored, i.e that the kinesin heads cooperate in moving along the microtubule.

Subsequent experiments by Svoboda and Block (1994) gave a significantly different result. Using optical trapping interferometry (Section 4.7) for calibration, they found a maximum force of

$$5\text{-}6 \text{ pN}.$$

Finally, Kojima et al. (1997), after widely varying the physicochemical parameters, found a limiting value of

$$8\text{-}9 \text{ pN}.$$

Several explanations for this disagreement were given. One reason may be that one experiment used GTP while the other used ATP as the energy source. The inconsistency may also be due to the different calibration methods or the different kinesin preparations employed. Finally, similarly as for myosin (see below), the force during a single stroke of kinesin may go through a maximum at different relative orientation of the kinesin head. A technique measuring the average force will then yield a lower result than a technique measuring essentially the force maximum.

Step width is also under investigation. Svoboda et al. (1993) have found a considerable statistical fluctuation of this value and Coppin et al. (1996) have shown that steps as short as 5 nm are possible. Nevertheless, the majority of step widths appears to be 8 nm, a value corroborated by the structure of the kinesin molecule, which has a 7-nm elongated part with a head which may cause the motion. Schnitzer and Block (1997) showed, using optical tweezers, that a single kinesin molecule uses a single ATP molecule per 8-nm step.

The kinetics of force generation by individual kinesin molecules has been measured by a combination of optical tweezers and UV microbeam (Higuchi, 1997). These experiments used the fact that kinesin needs ATP. The latter was present in an inactive form, as a caged compound. Only after a short UV laser pulse, is ATP liberated from its cage and becomes available for the kinesin. This is the start signal for the kinesin molecule to travel along the microtubule in 8 nm steps. The stroke frequency was dependent on the amount of ATP released: At an ATP concentration of 18 µmol/l, it took, on the average, 79 µs to recover and be prepared for the next stroke. At 90 mmol/l, the repetition frequency was faster, every 45 ms and at 450 µmol/l, the time from stroke to stroke was 31 ms. Slightly different values (159 ms at 10 mmol/l ATP and 38 ms at 1 mmol/l) were reported by Kojima et al. 1997.

A detailed study using modified kinesins by Inoue et al. (1997) showed that kinesin variants with a short flexible neck work as well as do native kinesin variants with a long neck (similar step width, similar speed), but that kinesins without a flexible neck show only poor performance.

### 4.3.4 Dynein – not as exact as kinesin

Dynein, as well as kinesin, is a motor protein working on microtubules. It directs minus end movement and, in the axons of nerves, retrograde (towards cell body) and slow anterograde (towards nerve tip) transport of vesicular material. In order to ascertain similarities and differences between these two motor molecules, dynein and kinesin (prepared from chicken embryo brains, kinesin also from squid brain) were used in the experiment described in the following. Since for kinesin experimental details have already been discussed in Section 5.4.2, only the experimental details for dynein will be described. Dynein was coupled to 143-nm-diameter latex beads at different bead/dynein molecule ratios. These ratios could be adjusted by a corresponding composition of the reaction mixture when dynein was bound to the beads. Several tests were used to show that in some experiments only one or very few dynein molecules were bound to the beads. When dynein-coated beads were added to microtubules previously fixed on microscope slides, three different types of beads could be observed:

1    beads moving irregularly (diffusing freely),
2    beads moving in a linear fashion, and
3    beads moving linearly and then abruptly dislocating themselves
     perpendicularly to the original direction of motion (off axis jumps).

The irregularly moving beads were just beads not bound to microtubules. The second group had bound and was transported on long microtubule filaments, the third group occasionally jumped from one microtubule filament to the next oriented approximately parallel to the former. In order to increase the number of beads on microtubules they were optically trapped by a titanium sapphire laser at a wavelength of 785 nm.

For quantitative evaluation the movement was observed by differential interference contrast microscopy (DIC) at high magnification and recorded on video tape with 30 pictures per second, i.e. with one picture every 33 milliseconds (Wang et al., 1995). At maximum magnification, one pixel in the video frame corresponds to 42 nm x 34 nm. By comparing two subsequent digitized video frames and using a special mathematical algorithm, fixed beads could be localized with an accuracy of better than 1nm (!). The accuracy of localization of dynein-coated beads bound to microtubules was approximately 6 nm. One reason for this poorer accuracy is that the 143-nm-diameter bead is not absolutely fixed by the 25-nm-diameter microtubule. In a sense the microtubule acts as a somewhat flexible track.

When compared with kinesin, it turns out that dynein is less exact. When kinesin is on its microtubule track, it moves forward and changes tracks less than once per micrometer. Only very occasionally does it stop or briefly reverse its direction. In contrast, dynein jumps from one microtubule protofilament to the next (i.e. it changes tracks) 5.1 times per micrometer. Since this type of movement is similar to that of a degenerated kinesin, which has only one motor head instead of two, one conclusion to be drawn from the work described here is that dynein might usually generate motion only with one head while intact kinesin is using two heads in a type of hand over model, where at least one head has contact to the microtubule at any given time.

## 4.3.5 Myosin/actin: Single heads can do the work

Myosin is the best-studied motor molecules. Much information has been obtained from experiments on whole muscle fibers. Also, a single molecule technique using a microneedle is available. Two types of fragment can be prepared from myosin: subfragment S1 with one head and heavy meromyosin (HMM) with two heads. Optical tweezers have been employed to compare the two.

### Box 54: Subjects of recent research (not all entailing the use of optical tweezers)

1. Does single-headed S1 produce the same force and displacement as HMM?
2. What is the force and displacement produced by HMM interacting with actins of different structure?
3. Is the slower F-actin sliding velocity measured in *in vitro* assays of wild type *Drosophila* and even due to a foreshortened work stroke or because of a lower cross bridge force?
4. Does S1 interact preferentially with actin monomers that have favorable orientation?
5. Is cross bridge detachment distortion independent?

In a typical optical tweezers experiment, an actin filament is coupled with its two ends to microbeads which are then held by a pair of optical tweezers. Myosin molecules are bound to a fixed support and try to shift the actin molecule. The force on the actin and its displacement during a stroke is sensed by a double beam optical trap. Since at high load the latter can be expected to be smaller than at a load close to zero, an electronic feedback mechanism is used to keep the load approximately constant, i.e. to obtain results at isometric conditions. The results of several experiments are summarized in Box 55.

As mentioned already in the section on kinesin, Ishijima et al. realized that the force development during a stroke is variable with a maximum of 5.9 pN and an

**Box 55: Force, stroke width and stiffness for one- and two-headed myosins as determined in different experiments.**

|              | Fin, M | Mol a S1    | Mol b S1  | Mol a HMM | Mol b HMM | Ishi M      |
|--------------|--------|-------------|-----------|-----------|-----------|-------------|
| Force        | 3-4 pN | 1.7 pN      | >1.7 pN   | 1.8 pN    | >1.7 pN   | 2.1–5.9 pN  |
| stroke width | 11 nm  | 15 nm       | (7.9 nm)  | 20 nm     | 4 nm*)    | 20 nm       |
| Stiffness    |        | 0.13 pN/nm  | <1 pN/nm  | <1 pN/nm  | 0.2 pN/nm |             |

| Fin M:                      | Finer et al., 1994, myosin                                    |
|-----------------------------|--------------------------------------------------------------|
| Mol a S1 and Mol a, HMM:    | Molloy et al., 1995 a with subfragment S1 and HMM            |
| Mol b S1 and Mol b, HMM:    | Molloy et al., 1995 b with subfragment S1 and HMM            |
| Ishi M:                     | Ishijima et al., 1996, myosin with glass needle, not tweezers |

*) large (up to 30 nm) forward and reverse (up to -25 nm) displacements were observed

average value of 2.1 pN. This may also partly explain the minor force variations in the other experiments. The differences in measured stroke widths may be due to different loads during force generation. Another possibility is that in the experiments reporting the large displacements a selection for large values due to better detectability took place.

## 4.3.6 Differences between skeletal and smooth muscle

So far, a quite important question on muscle function has not yet been addressed: the difference between skeletal and smooth muscle (as, for example, of the heart). Smooth muscles are slow. In vitro myosin propels actin molecules with only 10% of the speed observed in skeletal muscle. But smooth muscles produce 300 to 400% more force per myosin molecule or, more precisely, they produce the same force per cross sectional area as skeletal muscles, but a much smaller number (1/6) of myosin molecules. How can this be explained on the level of single myosin molecules?

Experiments using microneedles have already given some insight into the underlying mechanism. Optical tweezers (here not with the typical NdYAG laser at 1064 nm but with an NdYLF TFR laser at 1047 nm) were used to give a detailed answer (Guilford, 1997). The experimental strategy was similar as that used in the experiments described above. The result of these studies was that single myosin molecules from skeletal as well as from smooth muscle displaced their partner molecule actin by 11 nm and exerted 1.5. to 3.5 piconewton force per stroke. This suggests that an increased duty cycle (a higher stroke frequency), and not an increased force per stroke, is responsible for the differences between the two muscle types.

### 4.3.7 Molecular bungee: Titin

Actin acts as a sort of rail for myosin and the relative motion between actin and myosin is generating the muscle force. However, actin has to be elastically connected to the rigid parts of the muscle, the Z-membranes. The connecting molecule is titin or connexin. It consists of approximately 140 immunoglobulin domains andapproximately 1000 to 2000 amino-acid-long PEVK domains. The name of the latter comes from the fact that it is rich in proline (single letter code: P), glutamic acid (E), valine (V) and lysine (K). A single titin molecule can be fixed with its one end at the surface of a microscope slide or to a microbead which then is held by a micropipette. Its other side is naturally bound to myosin which in turn is coupled to a microbead. The whole system can be manipulated by calibrated optical tweezers.

At forces below 10 piconewtons, molecules can be reversibly stretched easily by 200 nm. This is interpreted as the reversible expansion of the PEVK domain by a factor of 1.8. At higher forces, a second structural transition indicates the stretching of the immunoglobulin domains. This process is reversible, but with a considerable temporal delay (hysteresis). Different forces required for this process have been reported by different working groups: 20 to 40 pN by Miklos et al. (1997) and 100 piconewtons by Tskhovrebova et al. (1997). A similar study using the calibrated tip of an atomic force microscope measured an even higher value: 150 to 300 piconewtons (Rief et al., 1997). The AFM experiments also give a hint where the discrepancies in the force values may come from: the measured force depends on the speed of pulling. This indicates that molecular forces cannot be regarded as static; when noncovalent bonds between single molecules are rupted this happens, simply stated, more by gliding under high friction than by a sort of cutting. Detailed atomic force microscopy data and their interpretation are available for the bond between streptavidin and biotin (Grubmüller et al., 1996). Also, by optical trapping experiments the breaking force for the bond between actin and skeletal muscle a-actinin has been measured to range from 1.4 to 44 piconewtons with an average value of 18 piconewtons (Miyata et al., 1996) and the variation has been interpreted as resulting from a dependence of the breaking force on the magnitude of the applied force.

In spite of the mentioned uncertainties it has become clear from these experiments that titin is designed to protect the muscle from overstretching. A slight overstretching of muscle will have no consequences since it is buffered by the reversible flexibility of the PEVK domains. A moderate overstretching has to be buffered by the immunoglobulin domains and this process is only reversible after some time. Finally, when the overstretching highly exceeds a few 100 piconewtons per titin molecule, things become irreversible and the muscle is hurt.

## 4.3.8 Laser microbeams for preparing the smallest functional unit of a muscle

While the study of single muscle motor proteins reveals fascinating details, the smallest physiologically functional unit is larger. The nitrogen laser microbeam (30–140 µJ, 3 ns pulse duration, up to 20 pulses per second) has allowed to isolate this minimal unit (3.5 µm x 28 µm), fragments of myofibrillar bundles (2.5 µm in diameter) and selected areas of myopathic fibers. The functional integrity of the myofibrillar bundle was checked by sudden release of caged calcium from nitrophen 7 which caused contraction from a length of 3 µm to 2.3 µm. From thicker muscle fibers (70 mm in diameter), approx. 1% of the sarcolemma could be removed, still leaving the fiber in a physiologically intact state. As a further application, sarcolemma vesicles were fused in order to obtain large vesicles for electrophysiological studies.

Thus the laser microbeam helps to explicate to physiology while optical tweezers investigate muscle function on a single molecule level. A dream for the future is to bridge the gap and to learn how single molecules orchestrate their function to make muscles work. This would be an ideal field for the combined use of laser microbeams and optical tweezers.

Box 56 summarizes a number of possible microbeam experiments which can be conducted already now:

**Box 56: Experiments for bridging the gap from single molecules to physiology**

- skinning muscles
- perforation of the sarcolemma of skeletal muscle fibres and removal of small patches of sarcolemma
- preparation and microdissection of fragments of myofibrillar bundles
- induction of fusion of sarcolemma vesicles
- inducing $Ca^{2+}$-dependent reactions by flash photolysis

## Summary and outlook

The forces producing interactions of myosin with actin or kinesin/dynein with microtubuli can be measured on a single molecule basis, when calibrated optical tweezers are used. Such forces are in the range of a few piconewtons.

These experiments lend themselves well to the use of microtools since one of the partners is a non-covalent polymer of individual protein molecules – actin is a polymer of G-actin and microtubuli are polymers of tubulins. We are now ready to proceed even further – to measure individual molecules of DNA.

## Selected literature

a) Kinesin

S.M. Block, L.R.S. Goldstein and B.J. Schnapp (1990) Bead movement by single kinesin molecules studied with optical tweezers. Nature 348, 348–352.

C.M. Coppin, J.T. Finer, J.B. Spudich and R.D. Vale (1996) Detection of sub-8nm-movements of kinesin by high resolution optical-trap-microscopy. Proc. Natl. Acad. Sci. 1913–1917.

H. Higuchi, E. Muto, Y. Inoue, T. Yanagida (1997) Kinetics of force generation by single kinesin molecules activated by laser photolysis of caged ATP. Proc. Natl. Acad. Sci. 94, 4395–4400.

Y. Inoue, Y.Y. Toyoshima, A.H. Iwane, S. Morimoto, H. Higuchi and T. Yanagida (1997) Movements of truncated kinesin fragments with a short or an arificial flexible neck. Proc. Natl. Acad. Sci. 7275-7280.

H. Kojima, E. Muto, H. Higuchi and T. Yanagida (1997) Mechanics of single kinesin molecules measured by optical trapping nanometry. Bioph. J. 73, 2012–2022.

S.C. Kuo and M.P. Sheetz (1993) Force of single kinesin molecules measured with optical tweezers, see also: R.D. Vale Measuring single protein motors at work, ibid. Science 260, 232-234.

M.J. Schnitzer and S.M. Block (1997) Kinesin hydrolyses one ATP per 8 nm step. Nature 389, 387–390.

K. Svoboda,, C.F. Schmidt, B.J. Schnapp and S.M. Block (1993) Direct observation of kinesin stepping by optical trapping interferometry. Nature 365, 721–727.

K. Svoboda and S.M. Block (1994) Force and velocity measurement for single kinesin molecules. Cell 77, 773–784.

b) Myosin

J.F. Finer, R.M. Simmons and J.A. Spudich (1994) Single molecule mechanics: piconewton forces and nanometer steps. Nature 368, 113–119.

W.H. Guilford, D.E. Dupuis, G. Kennedy, J. Wu, J.B. Patlak and D.M. Warshaw
(1997) Smooth muscle and skeletal muscle myosins produce similar unitary
forces and displacements in the laser trap. Bioph. J. 72.3, 1006–1021.

J.E. Molloy, J.E. Burns, J.C. Sparrow, R.T. Tregear, J. Kendrick-Jones and D.C.S.
White (1995) Single molecule mechanics of heavy meromyosin and S1 interacting with rabbit or *Drosophila* actins using optical tweezers. Bioph. J. 68,
298a–305a.

J.E. Molloy, J.E. Burns, J. Kendrick-Jones, R.T. Tregear and D.C.S. White (1995)
Movement and force produced by a single myosin head. Nature 378, 209–212.

A. Ishijima, H. Kojima, H. Higuchi, Y. Harada, T. Funatsu and T. Yanagida (1996)
Multiple- and single molecule analysis of the actomyosin motor by nanometre-
piconewton manipulation with a microneedle: Unitary steps and forces. Bioph.
J. 70, 383–400.

c) Dynein

A. Ashkin, K. Schütze, J.M. Dziedzic, U. Eutenauer and M. Schliwa (1990) Force
generation of organelle transport measured in vivo by an infrared laser trap. Nature 348, 346-348.

Z. Wang, S. Khan and M.P. Sheetz (1995) Single cytoplasmic dynein molecule
movement: Characterization and comparison with kinesin. Bioph. J. 69.5,
2011–2023.

d) Titin

S. Miklos, Z. Kellermayer, S.B. Smith, H.L. Granzier and C. Bustamante (1997)
Science 276., 1112–1116.

M. Rief, M. Gautel, F. Oesterhelt, J.M. Fernandez and H.E. Gaub (1997) Reversible unfolding of individual titin immunoglobulin domains by AFM. Science 276, 1109–1112.

L. Tshkovrebova, J. Trinick, J.A. Sleep and R.M. Simmons (1997) Elasticity and unfolding of single molecules of the giant muscle protein titin. Nature 387, 308–312.

## e) Others

H. Grubmüller, B. Heymann and P. Tavan (1996) Ligand binding: molecular mechanics calculation of the streptavidin-biotin ruption force. Science 271, 997-
999.

H. Miyata, R. Yasuda and K. Kinosita jr. (1996) Strength and lifetime of the bond
between acitn and skelatal muscle alpha – actinin studied with an optical trapping technique. Bioch. Bioph. Acta 1290, 83–88.

C. Veigel, R. Wiegand Steubing, A. Harim, C. Weber, K.O. Greulich and R.H.A.
Fink (1994) New cell biological applications of the laser microbeam technique:
the microdissection and skinning of muscle fibers and the perforation of sarcolemma vesicles. Eur. J. Cell. Biol. 140–148.

# 5 DNA as a molecular individuum

## 5.1 The ultimate DNA analytics: Single molecules

Probably the most prominent macromolecule of our time is the DNA molecule. At least, it is a hot candidate. The genome projects, which are essentially DNA sequencing projects, underpin its importance. DNA is responsible for the fact that we are all individuals – and you will learn soon how far the individuality of DNA molecules goes. Essentially, each single naturally occurring DNA molecule is different from all others. This is the reason why more and more scientists try to develop techniques for single DNA molecule analysis. You may have already guessed it: laser microbeams and optical tweezers play an important role.

### Box 57: DNA and RNA: Some textbook information

Chemically, DNA is a polymer of four different building blocks. Each monomer is a nucleotide, or in other words, a nucleoside triphosphate. The nucleosides, are organic bases bound with deoxyribose. Four different organic bases are involved in forming DNA. This box gives some basic information on DNA as you may find it in any textbook on molecular biology. The four organic bases and the corresponding nucleosides with their single letter code are as follows:

| Organic base | Nucleoside single | Letter code |
| --- | --- | --- |
| Adenine | Adenosin | A |
| Guanine | Guanosine | G |
| Cytosin | Cytidine | C |
| Thymine | Thymidine | T |

A and G are purine bases or purine nucleosides, respectively. Purines are combinations of a six ring (benzene-like) and a five ring. C and T are pyrimidines, consisting of six ring only. For the non-biochemist the nomenclature is puzzling. The following mnemonic hint is simplistic, but quit often useful:

*P**y**rimidines have a **y** in their name.*

A single strand of DNA is in a sense, hungry. It aims to form a double strand by pairing with a type of mirror image. The rules are surprisingly simple:

Purines pair only with pyrimidines and vice versa.

In most cases this simple rule is even more simplified. There are essentially only two pairs (known as the Watson-Crick pairs):

A pairs with T and vice versa
G pairs with C and vice versa

Again a mnemonic aid:

*round* letters pair with *round* letters.

There are deviations from this rule. But they will play no significant role in this book.
It is this tendency of pairing which makes DNA the blueprint of life. One single molecule strand may, by collecting pairing partners, become the template for a second molecule which pairs with the strand. This molecule is often called the complementary strand. In some sense it is the mirror image of the strand. While the complementary strand has, according to the Watson-Crick pairing mentioned above, a sequence of letters different from the strand, the information content is the same, since there is a 1:1 correlation, which may be changed only by reading errors.

## 5.1.1 DNA: Astronomical dimensions and unlimited variability

Chemically, DNA is a linear polymer consisting of four building blocks, the DNA bases. More specifically it is a polyanion, since each building block is negatively charged. In solution there is often a cloud of counterions arranged along the DNA molecules and in total the DNA with its counterions is electrically neutral. Its diameter in approximately 2 nm. Probably you are aware of the fact that a DNA molecule is very long. But do you really know how long it is? The answer is truly surpprising: each cell of your body contains approximately two meters of DNA – as a thin filament which is ingeniously packed in order to fit into a micrometer-sized cell nucleus without coiling up irreversibly. When you calculate how long the DNA of your own body is, you will end up with a second surprise. The DNA molecules of your body are long enough to span not just miles or even continents – they are long enough to cover the distance from Earth to Sun more than 100 times. So you should measure the total length of your DNA in light years or at least light hours rather than in miles. If you don't believe this, Box 58 shows you how to do the calculation. And when you go to Box 58 you will find another surprising result: the mass of the whole universe is not sufficient to synthesize one single copy of each possible DNA molecule with 120 bases in length – not really a very long molecule.

You may already surmise why this is discussed in a book on laser microtechniques. The reason is that the variability of DNA is virtually unlimited. Sequencing the whole human genome within a decade or so is a terribly slow process. In order to get at least a glimpse of the variability, we need much faster single molecule analytical techniques – even when they provide much less detailed information on a molecule than sequencing. Laser microtechniques may become useful tools for preparing such single molecules. This will be the subject of the following chapters.

### Box 58: Detailed calculation of length and variability of DNA molecules

The double-stranded DNA of each human cell contains 3 to $3.5 \cdot 10^9$ base pairs of the Watson-Crick type (see, for example, box 57. The distance from base pair to base pair is 3 Angstroms (0.3 nm)). Multiplication of both figures gives a length of approximately 1 m. This has to be doubled, since each human cell contains at least two sets of DNA, one inherited from the mother, one from the father. Thus, as an estimate we have

*2 m of DNA per human cell.*

The human body consists of approximately $10^{13}$ cells (See Box 39 in Section 3.2.3). Multiplying of the cell number with the DNA length gives $2 \cdot 10^{13}$ m DNA in the body of each human individual. Since 150000000 km (= 8 light minutes) is the distance between Sun and Earth, this corresponds to 130 of such distances, or 0.72 light days. In other words, we have the following surprising equivalence:

*The DNA of approx. 500 human individuals spans one light year.*

While the length of DNA molecules is in fact astronomical, the diameter is small: approximately 2 nm.

If we ask for the sequence variability of DNA we end up with the second surprise: the principal variability of, for example, DNA of the length of human DNA is far beyond anything we can imagine. Therefore, we try to tackle a much simpler problem: we ask how many different DNA molecules with a length of only 120 base pairs are possible, and how much material we need to synthesize just one exemplar of all of these molecules. For molecules of length 1 we have four possibilities: A C T G. For molecules of length 2 we have $4^2=16$ possibilities, AA, AC, AG, AT, CA, CC ....

*For all molecules with length 120 base pairs, there exist $4^{120}=10^{72}$ possibilities.*

Since 1 mol is $6 \cdot 10^{23}$ molecules this is $1.6 \cdot 10^{48}$ mol. The molecular weight of a basepair is 700 g. Molecules with 120 base pairs have a weight of 84 kg per mole. Thus $1.6 \cdot 10^{48}$ mol is

$$100 \cdot 10^{46} \text{ kg} = 2.5 \cdot 10^{19} \text{ masses of the Sun.}$$

In conclusion

*more than the visible mass of the Universe*

would be needed to synthesize one single molecule of each possible variants of a DNA molecule with 120 bases.

## 5.1.2 Handling of DNA

In order to handle and manipulate individual DNA molecules they are often coupled to micrometer-sized beads which act as a handle (for coupling, see also Box 63 in Section 5.2.2). With a trapped bead the DNA molecule can be manipulated with high spatial and temporal accuracy. For example, an individual DNA molecule can be stretched by viscous drag (see also Box 30 in Section 2.6.1) by pulling it through the solution. An even better control is achieved when the bead is held by the optical tweezers and electric fields are employed. Fig. 22 (from Hoyer et al., 1996) shows the stretching of a DNA in such a field.

An even finer control is possible. When the polarity of the electrostatic field is reversed the single DNA molecule can be rotated in solution.

In the experiments described so far there has been some uncertainty as to whether indeed single DNA molecules are seen. If the DNA tends to collapse as

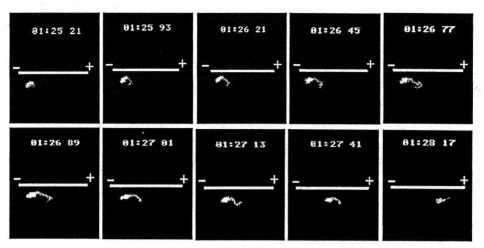

**Fig. 22:** *From top left to bottom right: collapsed DNA becomes increasingly stretched by the electrostatic field. At time 00:15:76 the field is switched off and the DNA collapses back onto the bead.*

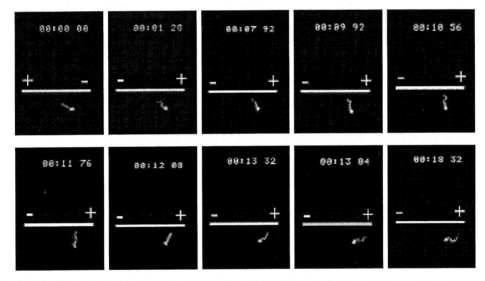

**Fig. 23:** *The bead is held by optical tweezers. The DNA molecule is directed towards the positive pole of the electrostatic field. When the field is reversed and subsequently slowly increased, the molecule changes its directions thus slowly rotating the bead. (From: Hoyer et al., 1996).*

was described above, there is also some chance that a number of molecules may aggregate, i.e. that bundles of molecules are seen. At least in Fig. 23 this may be a problem. While the aggregation of a few DNA molecules would not adversely affect principal ideas and results of the experiments, one would finally like to have greater assurance that indeed single molecules are seen.

163

## 5.1.3 Laser microdissection of single DNA molecules

Two types of DNA filaments are studied: Phage lambda DNA complexed with poly-L-lysine and naked DNA molecules. Two hours after staining, fluorescent particles were observed which differed in structure and color from fluorescent pollution. In order to confirm that the observed fluorescent particles indeed represent DNA, a number of tests were performed (Box 59). At least some tests mentioned in Box 59 strongly suggest that the filaments represent individual DNA molecules. We will try to provide further evidence in a three-stage process. First we use complexes of DNA with poly-L-lysine as models for chromosomal DNA. When during preparation of such complexes shearing is avoided by gentle mixing, multimolecular cables can be obtained, since the positively charged poly-L-lysine neutralizes repulsion between negatively charged DNA molecules.

Such a cable is shown in Fig. 24 (from Endlich et al., 1994). The ends of the cable have at least three different strands; i.e. in this case the strand of several molecules can be clearly identified.

For Fig. 25 a preparation protocol is used that is expected to yield individual molecules. Additionally, the tests in Box 59 support this finding.

**Box 59: Checklist for identifying single DNA molecules**

| Check | Result |
|---|---|
| Solution without DNA | No fluorescent particles |
| Restriction by EcoRI | Fluorescent particles disappear without indication of separate digestion of several molecules arranged side by side |
| Application of an electric field | Fluorescent particles do not disassemble during migration |
| Staining with ethidium bromide | Particles fluoresce orange |
| Additional staining with DAPI | Particles additionally fluoresce blue |
| Addition of $MgCl_2$ | Adhesion to the glass surface |
| Addition of poly-L-lysine | Condensation and fixation at the glass surface |
| Dynamical behavior of the particles | Condensation, translational movement, internal fluctuations without signs of disassembly |

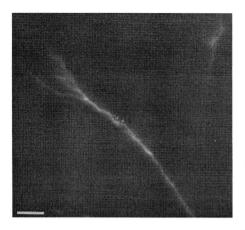

**Fig. 24:** *Cable of several DNA molecules. The DNA molecules in a cable can be distinguished from single molecules (Fig. 25) by their morphology.*

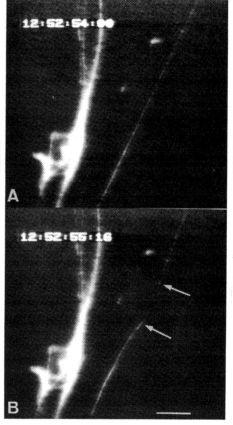

**Fig. 25:** *Laser microdissection of a single fluorescence stained DNA molecule fixed on the glass surface of the microscope slide. The bright object on the left is probably aggregated DNA.*

The background in Fig. 25 (from Endlich et al., 1994) is much higher than in Fig. 24 since the filament had a much lower fluorescence per length and, therefore, the sensitivity of the video camera had to be extended to its maximum value.

For the sake of greater certainty, DNA of Fig.25 was compared with DNA prepared almost identically as for electron microscopy, except for some steps specific to this latter technique. In fact, single DNA molecules were seen. This provided further evidence that the preparation technique is suitable for the purpose of these experiments.

## 5.1.4 The elasticity of a single DNA molecule

A long-discussed problem of polymer research is, how a flexible filamentous macromolecule migrates in an environment of high viscosity such as a gel. The problem is important, for example, to the understanding of electrophoresis. A particular aspect is the migration of a linear macromolecule in a high concentration of macromolecules of the same type, for example the migration of DNA in a high concentration of DNA molecules. This can be studied in a light microscope on a single molecule basis by fluorescently labeling a few molecules (the test molecules) while all other DNA molecules are not observable but comprise the viscous background (Perkins et al., 1994 a and b). This system is a model for three different physicochemical situations, depending on the time scale:

1 On a very short timescale the situation is comparable to a glass. Any perturbation will relax only gradually.
2 On an intermediate time scale the system behaves like rubber. Perturbations are transferred to a large environment.
3 On a very long time scale any pertubation can relax, i.e. the system behaves like a liquid.

These three definitions are valid for many systems. The basic problem is to find out which timescale is, in this sense, short, intermediate and long, and to find ways to perform an experiment within such scales. This is exactly where optical tweezers come onto the stage (Perkins et al., 1994 a and b; Quake et al., 1997; Smith and Chu, 1998).

Without optical tweezers it is possible to study solely the passive (thermal) motion of such an individual DNA molecule or the very directed motion in an electric field. In contrast, with optical tweezers any type of motion can be generated, at a wide range of speeds. Also, geometrically complex paths are possible.

This allows one to test a specific model for the motion of the test molecule through the background molecules. The model postulates imaginary tubes through which the test molecule can move (the reptation model). Lambda phage DNA molecules (48 kb or, correspondingly, 16 μm in length are used as background molecules. Lambda phage DNA is also used as test molecule. Now 5 or 6 of such molecules are linked together in order to give a molecule approximately 80 μm in length. Such a linked DNA molecule is particularly simple to obtain, since lamb-

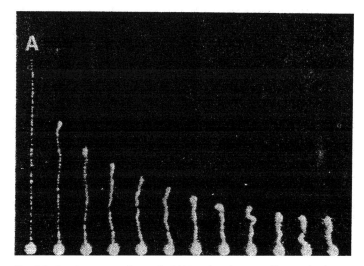

**Fig. 26:** *Condensation of a single DNA molecule originally stretched out by liquid flow. Reprinted from Perkins, 1994 b*

da phage, during its natural life cycle, programs the host cell to link its DNA. One can exploit this to get longer molecules. At the end of the test molecule a biotin labeled nucleic acid is incorporated. Such labeled DNA molecules are mixed with commercially available avidin-coated polystyrene microbeads of 1µm diameter. The avidin binds the biotin and thus the spheres bind the DNA test molecule. The beads and thus the test molecules are now pulled through the viscous background at different speeds, writing complex figures (which can be seen in the microscope since the DNA is fluorescently labeled). The fluorescence labeled DNA is extended by the viscous drag, which is higher at high pulling speed than at slow motion. Without viscous drag the test molecule relaxes. From the speed of relaxation it can be concluded that in fact the reptation model is valid for this type of motion.

In principle, the experiments decribed above characterize the properties of the background. The labeled DNA is just the test molecule with which the effects on the non visible background are visualized. In a second type of related experiments the elastic properties of the DNA molecule itself can be tested. The strategy is to stretch a long DNA molecule and exploit its natural tendency to collapse (relax) into a condensed, more globular form. Since the typical environment of DNA in many experiments is performed in buffer with a viscosity around 1 cPoise (see Box 30 in Section 2.6.1), is not highly viscous, the following experiment investigates DNA at this low viscosity. Unfortunately, under these conditions the tendency to relax is strong, and it is difficult to fully stretch a DNA molecule many tens of micrometers in length. After the flow has stopped, the relaxation of the DNA molecules can be observed. Fig. 26 shows the relaxation of a 39 μm long DNA molecule.

The same molecule is shown 12 times (drawn into the same figure) at 4.5.-second-intervals. On the very left side the molecule is extended so much that its fluorescence can hardly be seen. After 4.5 sec, at the end opposite from the microbead, a small bead like structure is seen. It is DNA which has locally condensed from the end of the molecule. By continuing condensation more of the molecule can be seen. Finally the molecule is much thicker, but reduced in length by a factor of more than 5 (7.7 μm as compared to originally 39.1 nm). The time progression of this condensation can be analyzed quantitatively using a microscope image analysis system. The relaxation follows an exponential law with a relaxation time $l_t$, which depends on the total length of the molecule according to

$$\lambda_t = L^{1.65 \pm 0.13} \approx L^{5/3}. \quad (35)$$

## 5.1.5 Two types of elasticity in DNA

The flexibility of the DNA molecule as you have seen it in the previous chapters has sparked interest to measure quantitatively the forces involved in DNA stretching. Several different techniques have been used for such experiments, for example, stretching DNA with the receding meniscus of a microscopic droplet of solution (Bensimon et al., 1995), binding a DNA molecule to a bead (see Box 63 in Section 5.2.2) and manipulating the latter micromechanically (Cluzel et al., 1996) or in a magnetic field (Strick et al., 1996). Finally, optical tweezers were used by the groups of Bustamante (Smith et al., 1996) and Block (Wang et al., 1997). In the experiments using optical tweezers force calibration was performed as described in Section 2.6.

In most of these experiments the force required for a given length expansion of single DNA molecule was measured. In the experiment by Smith et al. (1996) a double-stranded lambda phage DNA molecule could be expanded to its contour length (see Box 60) of approximately 15 μm with forces of a few piconewtons. After that, forces up to 65 piconewtons were not able to expand the molecule further. Everybody would have expected that the molecule would be rupted or deformed inelastically and irreversibly. Above 65 piconewtons, within a narrow range of 2 piconewtons, the DNA molecule revealed a new type of elasticity, i.e. there was again a linear relationship between force and extension. The narrow force range indicates a highly cooperative transition. The new elasticity prevailed up to an extension to 170% of the molecule's original contour length. The authors termed this type of DNA structure "S-DNA". As long as no forces above 100 piconewtons were applied, it was a completely reversible process, though with some temporal delay (hysteresis) when the the force was released and S-DNA was allowed to return back to the B-DNA state. For one given molecule, the process was reproducible several times. However, for a different lambda phage DNA molecule, the parameters, for example the force at which the transition from B-DNA to S-DNA occurred, were different and could be as low as 40 piconewtons. Whether this is some poorly understood irreproducibility or reflects the individuality of single DNA molecules remains to be seen.

### Box 60: End to end distance, contour length and persistence length

Defining lengths of macromolecules is similar to measuring distances of, for example, geographic sites on a map. The shortest distance (as the crow flies) is shorter than the distance you actually have to travel on the road.

In a similar way, macromolecules in solution are not straight, but curved (coiled). You may be interested in its

"end to end distance"

(equivalent to the air distance in geography) or you may be interested in the true length of the molecule, its

"contour length".

For many molecules the end to end distance is the square root of the contour length, but not always.

For some purposes flexible macromolecules can be imagined as being composed of stiff straight rods connected by hinges which allow the coiling. The length of these virtual rods is called

"persistence length".

The latter is dependent on a number of physicochemical parameters such as salt concentration (ionic strength) or on the presence of substances binding to DNA (particularly molecules fitting exactly between the steps of the DNA ladder (intercalators).

Various physicochemical parameters such as the ionic strength have a significant influence on the structural data of DNA (Baumann et al., 1997). In sufficiently high concentrations of monovalent salt cations such as $Na^+$ the persistence length of double-stranded DNA saturates at approximately 45 to 50 nm. Multivalent ions can reduce the persistence length to 25 to 30 nm and it makes a difference, if the charge in these cations is concentrated such as in $Mg^{++}$, or spatially distributed such as in putrescine or spermidine.

The single molecule experiments described so far all used lambda phage DNA with a contour length of approximately 15 μm. Even longer DNA constructs were used. Block's group (Wang et al. 1997) improved the trapping technique further. DNA molecules as short as 1 μm, corresponding to approximately 3 kilobases can now been measured. This is a significant improvement since now plasmid-sized DNA molecules can be investigated. The experimental data, similar to those reported by Bustamante's group, were evaluated with four different theoretical models which all involve the contour length. Three "worm-like chain" models gave quite good fit values when a persistence length of 47 nm (138 base pairs) was used.

In the experiments of Smith et al. (1996, see above), in addition to double-stranded DNA, single-stranded DNA was investigated. The persistance length was measured to be only 0.75 nm, i.e. two bases (instead of 138 bases for double-stranded DNA), indicating virtually total flexibility of the single-stranded DNA.

## Summary and outlook

The almost unlimited variability of DNA can be fully understood only when true single molecule techniques are employed. Laser microbeams and optical tweezers offer such a possibility. When DNA has to be trimmed with micrometer accuracy to a preselected size this is possible with the laser microbeam. No sequence-specific restriction sites are needed. After coupling DNA to micrometer sized beads, one has full spatial control over individual DNA molecules. The experiments on the flexibility of individual DNA molecules have revealed details which were hardly detectable in bulk experiments, since in the latter the different structural transitions probably would have been observed simultaneously and therefore a sort of intermediate transition would have been seen.

## Selected literature

C.G. Baumann, S.B. Smith, V.A. Bloomfield and C. Bustamante (1997) Ionic effects on the elasticity of single DNA molecules. Proc. Natl. Acad. Sci. 94.12, 6185–6190.

D. Bensimon, A. Simon, V. Croquette and A. Bensimon (1995) Stretching DNA with a receding meniscus: experiments and models. Phys. Rev. Lett. 74, 4754-4757.

P. Cluzel, A. Lebrun, C. Heller, R. Lavery, J.L. Viovy. D. Chatenay and F. Caron (1996) DNA: An extensible molecule. Science 271, 792–794.

N. Endlich, A. Harim and K.O. Greulich (1994) Microdissection of single DNA molecules and DNA-polycation complexes with a UV laser microbeam in a classical light microscope. Exp. Tech. Phys. 40.1, 87-93.

N. Endlich, C. Hoyer, A. Harim, S. Monajembashi and K.O.Greulich (1996) Special issue on single molecule detection: Micromanipulation of single DNA molecules by laser microbeam and optical tweezers. Exp. Tech. Phys. 41.2, 303–311.

C. Hoyer, S. Monajembashi and K.O. Greulich (1996) The combined optical, electrostatic and enzymatic handling of single DNA molecules. Progress in Biomedical Optics, paper 2928-33.

C. Hoyer, S. Monajembashi and K.O. Greulich (1996) Laser manipulation and UV induced single molecule reactions of individual DNA molecules. Biotech. J. 52.2, 65–73.

T.T. Perkins. D.E. Smith and S. Chu (1994a) Direct observation of tube like motion of a single polymer chain. Science 264, 819 –822.

T.T. Perkins. S.R. Quake, D.E. Smith and S. Chu (1994b) Relaxation of a single DNA molecule observed by optical microscopy. Science 264, 822–826.

S.R. Quake, H. Babcock and S.Chu (1997) The dynamics of partially extended single molecules of DNA. Nature 388, 151–154.

D. E. Smith, S. Chu (1998) Response of flexible polymers to a sudden elongational flow Science 281, 1335–1340.

S.B. Smith, Y. Cui and C. Bustamente (1996) Overstretching B-DNA: The elastic response of individual double stranded and single stranded DNA molecules. Science 271, 795–799.

T.R. Strick, J.F. Allemand, D. Bensimon, A. Bensimon and V. Croquette (1996) The elasticity of a single supercoiled DNA molecule. Science 271, 1835–1837.

M.D. Wang, H. Yin, R. Landick, J. Gelles and S.M. Block (1997) Stretching DNA with optical tweezers, Bioph. J. 72.3, 1335–1346.

# 5.2 Single molecule DNA reactions

With the two experiments described in the next few pages we are approaching the ultimate limit of microtool sensitivity: Reactions of single enzyme molecules with single DNA molecules. Again, optical tweezers will play an important role.

## 5.2.1 From general properties to single molecule reactions

Enzyme reactions with DNA or RNA molecules are central to molecular biology. The following enzyme types are particularly important:

- Exonucleases
- (Restriction-) Endonucleases
- DNA and RNA Polymerases
- Ligases
- Phosphoylases, Methylases

**Box 61: Properties of DNA-Exonuclease from *E. coli***

The nucleases degrade DNA. Exonucleases cut (digest) it from the the start of the sequence (which is the called the 5′ end) or from the 3′ end. The terminology comes from the chemistry of DNA and will not be discussed further here. The digestion products may be mono- or oligonucleotides. There exist exonucleases acting only on single strands or only on double strands and some enzymes act on both forms of DNA.
A set of exonucleases, all isolated from *E. coli* bacteria, is on the market:

| Exonuclease | Type of DNA | Direction | Major products |
|---|---|---|---|
| I | ss DNA | 3′→5′ | mononucleotides |
| III | ds DNA | 3′→5′ | mononucleotides |
| V | ss and ds DNA | both directions | oligonucleotides |
| VII | ss DNA | both directions | oligonucleotides |
| VIII | ss and ds DNA | 5′→3′ | mononucleotides |

## Box 62: Endonuclaeses

Endonucleases cut a long DNA molecule in several still comparatively long pieces. The names of these enzymes usually consist of an abbreviation of the organism from which they are isolated and a running number. For example, the restriction endonucleases EcoR1 to EcoR5 are derived from the coli bacterium *Escherichia coli*. R1 is the first restriction enzyme detected; R5 is the fifth one. Restriction endonucleases recognize short sequences of DNA, bind there and cut exactly in, or close to, this sequence. Presently, some 200 restriction endonucleases with recognition sites from four up to eight bases are known. The probability with which a long piece of DNA can be cut by restriction endonucleases, or rather the average length of the resulting DNA pieces after cutting (after restriction) can be roughly estimated from the size of the recognition site. Since a given sequence of six bases occurs with the statistical probability of $1:4^6=1:4096$, the expected length should be approx. of this order. This is not quite the case, however, since DNA sequences are not statisticallly arranged but have to code for proteins. For example, the DNA of prokaryotes is often rich in the bases A and T while, particularly the coding regions of higher organisms, are rich in the bases G and C. Thus there are deviations from the purely statistical estimates. The table below lists several restriction endonucleases, their cutting sites and their number of sites found in the 4.2 megabases of the genome of *Escherichia coli* (Karlin et al., 1992).

| | | |
|---|---|---|
| Bam H1 | GGATTC | 470 |
| Eco RI | GAATTC | 613 |
| Eco RV | GATATC | 1159 |
| Hind III | AAGCTT | 518 |
| Kpa I | GGTACC | 497 |
| Pst I | CTGCAG | 848 |
| Pvn II | CAGCTG | 1435 |
| Average | 7 enzymes | 791 |
| Theoretically 6 bases | 4200000/4096 | 1025 |
| Theoretically 7 bases | 4200000/16384 | 256 |
| Theoretically 8 bases | 4200000/65536 | 64 |

It is not too surprising that the experimental values for a coding DNA and the purely statistical theoretical values differ significantly. Nevertheless, none of the enzymes above has a frequency which could be mixed up with an enzyme with cutting sites of other lengths. Some cutting sites are systematically overrepresented. For example, cutting sites for the restriction endonuclease Alu (isolated from *Arthrobacter luteus*) occurs every 1000 base pairs in gene rich regions of the human genome.

When molecular biologists use them for modification of DNA they need information about the reaction mechanisms of these enzymes. Some of their bulk properties are known and summarized in various boxes of this chapter. A moderate degree of microheterogeneity can be detected by macroscopic experiments, for example, when an enzyme consists of two or three isoforms with differing kinetic constants. Such isoforms can, however, only be detected when they are present at least in an abundance of a few percent. Probably, on the single molecule basis a much larger heterogeneity prevails.

Reaction details resulting from the individuality of DNA sequences or from different enzyme molecules so far could not be studied. One may easily envision that true single molecule techniques will give unprecedented insights into the secrets of basic reactions of molecular biology.

## 5.2.2 Cutting of an individual DNA molecule by the restriction endonucleases Apa 1

The first single molecule restriction reaction which was observed in the light microscope was that of the endonuclease Apa 1. (Endlich et al., 1995; Hoyer et al., 1996). It has a six-base restriction site (GGGCC!C) and thus should statistically cut every 4096 bases. However, a specific target molecule, the 48 kb long DNA of lambda phage, was used. Since phage DNA is AT rich, one expects that the number of restriction sites is smaller than statistically calculated. In fact, lambda phage has only one restriction site for Apa 1 on its 15 µm long DNA molecule. The DNA molecule is coupled to a polystyrene microbead which acts as a handle for holding the molecule with the optical tweezers (see Box 63). Using this handle, the single DNA molecule can be transported from a distant site to the site of reaction in the visual field of the microscope. There, it can be held, fixed anywhere in the reaction droplet; one has complete spatial control over this single DNA molecule.

In the case of restriction of a single DNA molecule there is only a "yes" or "no" answer. In other word, the yield of the reaction is either 0% or 100%. Therefore the starting point of the restriction reaction has to be controlled. Thus, in addition to the above mentioned spatial control temporal, control is required.

For this purpose the $Mg^{2+}$-ions, essential for the endonuclease activity, are complexed. The caged compound of $Mg^{2+}$ with DM-nitrophen can be destroyed by UV-light (360 nm), the ions are liberated, the enzyme is activated and the reaction is started.

## Box 63: Coupling DNA to microbeads

The first step of the specific reaction is end-labelling of the lambda-phage DNA (New Eng-land Biolabs) by terminal transferase (Boehringer Mannheim, Germany) with dATP. The length of the resulting poly(A)-tail is between 50 and 150 nucleotides, depending on the duration of the transferase reaction. Subsequently a poly(T)$_{35}$-biotin molecule (Serva, Hei-delberg, Germany) is hybridized to the poly(A)-tail. Streptavidin labeled beads with 1 µm diameter (Polysciences, Germany) are used for the coupling reaction. The number of strep-tavidin molecules per bead and the binding capacity are not known. In order to obtain on-ly one DNA molecule per bead the DNA solution is diluted to a molecular ratio, beads:DNA = approx. 10:1. The result is one biotin molecule at each end of a lambda-phage DNA molecule. The streptavidin-labeled beads and the biotin-labeled lambda-phage molecules are mixed in a binding buffer (5 mM TrisHCl, 0,5 mM EDTA, 1 M NaCl). In order to prevent DNA from collapsing or adhesion to the glass surfaces and to see the trapping under physiological conditions the buffer has to be changed (8 mM TrisHCl, 0,8 mM EDTA, 2 mM NaCl 0,01% Tween) either by dialysis or by dilution. Finally the DNA is stained with DAPI (Hoechst, Germany). Before use, the DNA solution is heated to 65 °C for a few minutes, following the protocol of Perkins et al., 1994started.

## Box 64: Polymerases and ligases

*Polymerases* do the opposite of exonucleases: they read the blueprint DNA (the tem-plate) and synthesize a DNA macromolecule with a complementary sequence base by base. DNA polymerases use desoxribonucleotides as substrate and synthesis DNA. Cor-respondingly, RNA polymerases produce RNA. As with exonucleases their direction of synthesis is directed (see table below).

|  | Direction of synthesis | Number of subunits | Function |
|---|---|---|---|
| Polymerase I | 3'→5' and 5'→3' | 1 | DNA repair |
| Polymerase II | 3'→5' | 1 | SOS repair, i.e. DNA repair after catastrophic damage |
| Polymerase III | 3'→5' | 10 | DNA replication |

Polymerase III which is involved in DNA replication is much more complex (10 subunits) than the two other polymerases.

*Ligases* combine two DNA molecules. A requirement for such a ligation is that the two DNA molecules to be recombined fit each other; i.e. the need to have complementary ends. These ends can be produced by digesting (trimming) the two DNA molecules with suitable restriction endonucleases.

In Fig.27 the restriction can be observed 15.76 seconds after reaction start. The longer part of the DNA molecule drifts towards the positive pole of a moderate electric field. The shorter part collapses onto the microbead because of the free $Mg^{2+}$-ions being present after UV photolysis of the caged compound. Free Mg-ions are known to induce the compaction of DNA.

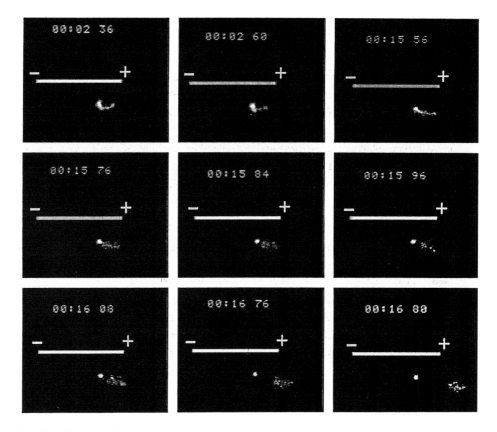

**Fig. 27:** *After 15.76, the restriction by Apa I is visible. One part of the molecule is pulled away and leaves the focus plane, therefore it becomes defocused, while the rest is still bound to the bead and remains in the trap. Scale bar 30 μm.*

## 5.2.3 Transcription against a force (Yin et al., 1995)

The experiment described below is to date probably the most sophisticated experiment performed on single molecules using optical tweezers. It investigates which force a single molecule of the enzyme RNA polymerase exerts when it reads DNA and how efficiently it does this. For the experiment, RNA polymerase from *E. coli* was used. For this enzyme an *in vitro* transcription assay, already developed earlier for other purposes, was used.

Such a molecule can be fixed to the cover glass surface of a flow cell for a microscope. When DNA and all essential components for *in vitro* transcription are present, the RNA polymerase will catch a DNA molecule, pull it through its active site and synthesize RNA with a sequence complementary to the sequence of the piece of DNA which was just read. When the DNA signals a stop codon the transcription is finished and the RNA falls off the polymerase. When a polystyrene microbead (0.52 µm diameter) is coupled to one end of the DNA which serves as a template, the bead will be pulled with the DNA towards the fixed RNA polymerase molecule. Nobody can say what will happen when the microbead approaches the RNA polymerase molecule. This was not experimentally tested. The strategy was different: the microbead at the end of the DNA molecule can be held in the center of the beam of calibrated optical tweezers of the type described in Section 2.6. The transcribing RNA polymerase tries to pull the DNA out of the tweezers, but with increasing distance from the tweezer's center the force increases. How far the bead can be displaced by the transcription process depends on the stiffness of the trap and the latter depends on the laser power. With a stiffness of 0.03 pN per nm, a displacement of 33 nm corresponds to 1 pN. The result of such an experiment is that *E. coli* RNA polymerase can pull with up to 14 pN. This result is surprising. For typical motor proteins a maximum force of 6 pN or less was found. Obviously it is a comparatively tough task to transcribe through DNA and therefore the polymerase must work harder than proteins driving a muscle with a total force production in the kilopond range.

Not only was it not possible to predict the absolute value of the force exerted by *E. coli* RNA polymerase; the efficiency with which it converts chemical into mechanical power could not be predicted either. The mechanical energy produced during the insertion of each single nucleotide into the nascent RNA can be calculated as force multiplied with distance. The latter is 0.34 nm, the final distance between nucleotides in the polymerized RNA. On the other hand, the chemical energy which is released by one reaction step is known from bulk experiments. The result is that for *E. coli* RNA polymerase under optimal physicochemical conditions

*the chemomechanical energy conversion rate is up to 42%.*

This compares well with the corresponding rates for the motor proteins kinesin and myosin (both up to 60%).

What is interesting in the context of this book is the fact that DNA does not run smoothly through the active site of such enzymes; there may be a type of friction between DNA and enzyme. Enzymes of the transcription machinery are the most powerful molecular motors known so far.

## Summary and outlook

At the sensitivity limits of biochemistry, when the reactions of single molecules are to be observed under the light microscope, optical tweezers are central tools. They can be used for handling the reaction partners and they can be used to exert and measure forces. So far, only a few experiments have been performed, but it can be envisioned that a large number of biochemical reactions will be studied in the future, for example reactions of the enzymes mentioned in Box 62 and Box 64. A particularly exciting aspect is the possiblity to assemble whole single molecule reaction chains with the help of optical tweezers.

## Selected literature

N. Endlich, C. Hoyer, A. Harim, S. Monajembashi and K.O. Greulich (1995) Micromanipulation of single DNA molecules by laser microbeam and optical tweezers. Exp. Tech. Phys. 41.2, 303–311.

C.Hoyer, S. Monajembashi and K.O. Greulich (1996) Laser manipulation and UV induced single molecule reactions of individual DNA molecules. J. Biotech. 52.2, 65–73.

S. Karlin, C. Burge and A.M. Campbell, (1992) Nucleic Acids Res. 20, 1363–1370.

T.T. Perkins. D.E. Smith and S. Chu (1994) Direct observation of tube like motion of a single polymer chain. Science 264, 819–822.

H. Yin, M.D. Wang, K. Svoboda, R. Landick, S.M. Block and J. Gelles (1995) Transcription against an applied force. Science 270, 1653–1656.

# 5.3 Intermezzo III: Genes, chromosomes and genetic diseases

The novelty in the DNA experiments described so far came primarily from the application of the laser microbeam, optical tweezers or the two together. Thus these experiments could be understood with comparatively little knowledge of molecular biotechnology or biomedicine. The following chapters will lead us into molecular genetics and cytogenetics. There, the laser microtools have a very simple task: cut and transport. The difficulty and sophistication of these experiments lies in the underlying molecular technology. In other words: here we have an example where interesting experiments can be performed and understood only by a combination of quite different fields of science. "Intermezzo III" summarizes some of the basic knowledge required to understand and interpret experiments described in the subsequent Section 5.4 on microdissection of chromosomes. As with the other "intermezzo" sections: if you are a biologist you may browse through Section 5.3 or skip it and immediately continue with Section 5.4.

## 5.3.1 Packing DNA: Chromatin

You know already that two DNA molecules (the one from the father and the one from the mother) of a human cell are each approximately 1 m long and that they have a diameter of 2 nm. They have to be packed into a cell nucleus of approximately 5 μm linear dimension. Try to imagine what this would mean in macroscopic terms: it is comparable to packing 1000 km of a 2-mm-thick thread into a room 5 m long, 5 m wide and 5 m high. When this is not done in a very careful and organized way there is probably only one word to describe the result: chaos! That's not exactly what a cell needs. In the cell the DNA has to be replicated with high fidelity between two cell divisions. And replication is only one task of DNA in a cell. It also has to be transcribed into RNA, which finally is translated into the working molecules of a cell, the proteins. For all of this, the DNA has to be made accessible to the enzyme machineries which are involved in replication and transcription This changes dramatically when the cell sets out to divide. Then the degree of packing is highly increased. You may easily imagine that it is essential for a cell to highly organize this interplay of packing and making DNA accessible. A schematic representation is given in Fig. 28.

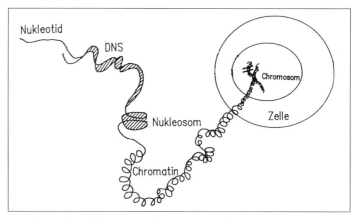

**Fig. 28:** *Packing of DNA into a chromosome. The scale increases from left to right.*

The human cell has solved this problem by using several levels of packing. The DNA double helix is wound around roughly cylindrical protein complexes, the nucleosomes, with linear dimensions of the order of 10 nm. Approximately 150 to 180 bases cover, in two complete loops, one nucleosome. Between one nucleosome and the next there are several tens of bases not covering a nucleosome, the linker. The whole structure looks like a string of beads of 10–12 nm thickness and is called the "low order structure" of chromatin. As if one were to wind a string of beads around the finger, the low order structure is packed further into a thicker structure, the high order structure. There is some discussion in the literature, as to whether this higher order structure is regular, for example a solenoid of 30 nm diameter, or if it is just caused by irregular aggregation of the nucleosomes. In any event, it allows for regular packing and unpacking.

At small salt concentrations (below 50 mM NaCl) the low order structure prevails while above 100 mM, particularly at the physiological salt concentration of 150 mM, the high order structure is favored.

## 5.3.2 From chromatin to chromosomes

The next higher degree of packing is not as well studied as the chromatin structural variants. One model hypothesizes that the high order structure itself is coiled into a type of hyper-helix with a diameter of the order of 100 nm and after a further, so far poorly defined, stage of packing an approximately cylindrical structure, the chromatid with a diameter of 1-2 μm, becomes visible in the microscope. The chromatid is one arm of a chromosome.

Since, in the whole process of DNA packaging described above, the diameter has increased by three orders of magnitude, in this grossly cylindrical symmetry the volume has increased by six orders of magnitude and it is now easily possible to pack the 2 m of human DNA into a nucleus with a few μm diameter.

A simple experiment gives insight into the poorly defined stage of the packaging process: A whole chromosome is held by glass microtools (optical tweezers would be too soft to do the job) and the chromosome is stretched. Then, fine structure can be recognized.

The 1 m long DNA molecule is partitioned into smaller sections which are separately packed into chromosomes of different size and different appearance. In human cells the two sets of DNA molecules are packed into 22 pairs of chromosomes which are numbered according to their size. The largest chromosome pair is called chromosome number 1, the second largest #2 and so forth. Chromosomes with high numbers are small. With the two smallest chromosomes, #21 and #22, a mistake was made when the chromosome numbers were first assigned. In actual fact, #21 is the smallest and #22 is a little bit larger. The 22 chromosomes coming in pairs are called the autosomes, each of the two members of the pair are called homologues. In addition to these 22 pairs of autosomes, each human cell has a pair of sex chromosomes. Females have two X chromosomes, one from the father and one from the mother. The size of the X chromosome is comparable to the size of chromosome #7. The male chromosome pair is XY, where the Y of course has to be inherted from the father. The Y chromosome is the smallest one and contains, among others, the SRY gene which in development of an embryo determines the sex.

Box 65 gives the physical size of selected human chromosomes in megabases. An interesting piece of information would be the density of genes on such chromosomes. This information is not yet available. However, there is a quantity which can probably be correlated with genes: sequence tagged sites (STSs). These are short sequence elements of which the localization on individual chromosomes is known. Since the STSs are derived from messenger RNA which had previously been transcribed, one assumes that they are related to genes.

**Box 65: Selected human chromosomes and the densitiy of sequence tagged sites**

| Chromosome | Megabases | STS density | Absolute STSs[*) |
|---|---|---|---|
| 1 | 248 | 1.4 | 347 |
| 7 | 161 | 1.1 | 177 |
| 12 | 135 | 1.0 | 135 |
| 13 | 92 | 0.6 | 55 |
| 19 | 63 | 2.6 | 164 |
| 21 | 37 | 0.8 | 30 |
| X | 155 | 0.6 | 93 |

[*) Megabases multiplied by STS density.
Table compiled from data given in T.J.Hudson et al., 1995

As can be seen from Box 65, human chromosome sizes vary by almost an order of magnitude. The STS densities vary by more than a factor of four. The small chromosome 19 contains almost the same number of STSs as the comparably large chromosome 7. Chromosome 21 is not only the smallest one (with the exception of the Y chromosome with 26 megabases) but has also a small STS density. This may be the reason why people with three instead of two chromosomes 21 survive, albeit with massive health problems (trisomy 21, Down`s syndrome, mongolism), while other trisomies cause prenatal death or early after birth (except multisomies of the well regulated X chromosome, see below)

The fact that different chromosomes have different STS densities may be interesting, for example when one plans a laser microdissection experiment (see Section 5.4) and is more interested in the technical development than in a specific chromosome. Then it might be useful to choose a chromosome rich in STSs since there the probability is higher to find something interesting than in a chromosome with poor STS density.

**Box 66: Some nomenclature from cytogenetics**

A normal human chromosome set is abbreviated as

46, XX (normal female) or 46, XY (normal male)

which indicates that 46 chromosomes are present, of which two are the sex chromosomes. XX in females and XY in males. Occasionally one finds

47, XXX or 48, XXXX or 49, XXXXX

These are females with one, two or three additional sex chromosomes. Since the activity of X chromosomes is particularly well regulated, such females are viable. Also, occasionally one finds

46, XX male

i.e. males with apparently two female sex chromosomes. More detailed examination in most cases shows that one of the X chromosomes has harbored the sex-determining region of the male chromosomes, i.e. the individual is only in cytogenetic but not in molecular-genetic terms a female. Before molecular DNA probes became available this caused problems in sex tests, for example, during sport events such as the Olympic games. The mere number of chromosomes is obviously not important for the phenotype of an organism. For example the reindeer-like animal "muntiac" whose number of DNA bases in its genome similar to that of man, has only five chromosome pairs. Also, the genome of rice has only a fifth of the DNA of that of maize but has 24 chromosomes as compared to 20 in the latter ( see also Box 68).

## 5.3.3 Banded chromosomes and cytogenetic nomenclature

The size of the individual human chromosomes (as well of chromosome sets of other organisms) is not sufficiently characteristic for them to be identified unambiguously. A first help can come from the fact that the human chromosomes from early metaphase have an appearance resembling the letter X. The crossover point is the centromere (see Intermezzo II). It can be located almost exactly in the center of the chromosome. Such symmetric chromosomes are called metacentric. The centromere can also be located close to one end. It is then called acrocentric. The mouse, for example, has mainly acrocentric chromosomes. The centromere divides the chromosome into a short arm (the p arm) and a long arm (the q arm). The ratio of long arm divided by the whole length of the chromosome is the centromere index. This quantity is an additional identification marker for chromosomes.

But even this is not sufficient to unequivocally identify the different chromosomes. Therefore, several staining methods have been developed which give the chromosomes a barcode-like appearance. The most widely used technique is the "Giemsa banding".

It turns out that the DNA in the dark bands is rich in the nucleotides A and T whereas the light bands are rich in G and C. Also, most active genes are found in the light bands. If genes in the dark bands are found they are often "household genes", i.e. genes which are needed by the cell for basic processes of life.

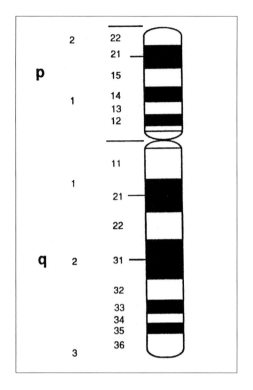

**Fig. 29:** *Schematic representation of a Giemsa-banded chromosome 7 with its p and q arm and its sub-bands.*

Bands are designated as follows: The band name consists of the number of the chromosome, the letter p or q, indicating if it is a band in the long or in the short arm, and a number which can be an integer for a coarse description or floating point for specific designation. A small number designates bands close to the centromer (central), a large number bands at the tips of the chromosome (distal). For example

$$7q35.1$$

is a band approximately in the middle of the long arm of chromosome 7. Fig. 29 shows schematically a Giemsa-banded chromosome 7.

## Box 67: Genes and gene sizes

Genes may have very different sizes. There are several reasons for this variability: on the one hand their gene products may be very different. On the other hand, the number of introns , i.e. sequence elements which are not used for coding, and the number of exons may be different. Introns are included when the gene size is given. The table summarizes some quantitative examples:

|  | Gene sizes |
| --- | --- |
| Dystrophin | > 2 Mb |
| Large genes | 60-100 kb |
| Medium sized genes | 40-50 kb |
| Vasopressin receptor | 6 kb |
| Smallest human genes | 2-3 kb |

1 kb means 1000 bases, 1 Mb means 1 million bases. The expressions kb and kbp, and Mb and Mbp respectively are equivalent. Kbp and Mbp are occasionally used when double-stranded DNA is discussed.

## 5.3.4 Genome sizes of different organisms

An organism's full complement of genes is called its genome. In order to understand the function of genomes it is important to know how many bases comprise a genome, how this information is packed into chromosomes and how effective the DNA is used to code for genes. The latter is often expressed as number of genes per million bases (megabase). Box 68 gives an overview.

## Box 68: Genome sizes of different organisms (modified from Collins 1995)

|  | Mega bases | Chromosomes | Genes | Genes per megabase |
| --- | --- | --- | --- | --- |
| Prokaryotes (cells without nucleus) |  |  |  |  |
| Mycoplasma genitalium | 0.5 |  | 482 | 950 |
| Haem. influenzae (bacterium) | 1.5 |  | 1700 | 1100 |
| Escherichia coli (coli-bacterium) | 4.2 |  | 4000 | 950 |

Eukaryotes (cells with nucleus)

| | | | | |
|---|---|---|---|---|
| Sacch.cerv. (yeast) | 15 | | 6000 | 400 |
| Arab.thaliana (plant) | 100 | | 25000 | 250 |
| Caen.elegans (worm) | 100 | | 13000 | 130 |
| Dros.melanogaster (fruitfly) | 120 | | 10000 | 83 |
| Mus musculus (mouse) | 3000 | | 80000 | 27 |
| Human | 3000 | 46 | 80000 | 27 |
| Human X chromosome | 200 | | | |
| Rice | 435 | 24 | | |
| Sorghum | 772 | 20 | | |
| Maize | 2509 | 20 | | |
| Barley | 5307 | 14 | | |
| Rye | 7623 | 14 | | |
| Wheat | 15970 | 42 | | |

The figures for the two first organisms are exact since these genomes have been sequenced. The others are estimates. Two further numbers can be calculated directly from the table using the following formulae:
The length l of the DNA is

$$l \text{ (in } \mu m) = 30000 \cdot \text{number of bases.} \quad (42)$$

The weight of the DNA is

$$w \text{ (in femtogram)} = 1 \text{ fg per megabase.}$$

Some of the major conclusions to be drawn from Box 68 are:

1 Approximately 0.5 megabases and 482 genes are needed to make the simplest organisms known so far.

2 Prokaryotes pack ca. 1000 genes into one megabase, i.e. they require on average 1000 bases per gene.

3 Simple organisms such as the roundworm, the fruit fly or the plantlet *Arabidopsis* require approximately 100 megabases (half the size of the human X chromosome) and 10000–20000 genes.

4 The genomes of mouse and man (and other mammals) are, in these terms, equal. Their number of genes is fourfold that of simple multicellulear organisms.

5 Plants as similar as rice and wheat differ by more than a factor of 30 in genome size.

### 5.3.5 Genetic diseases

Most human genes are error-tolerant, i.e. minor errors in the DNA sequence coding for a gene are without consequence for the organism. In some cases, however, even a single error in the DNA is disastrous. This is the case, for example, in carriers of sickle cell anemia or cystic fibrosis. In order to develop therapies against such diseases it is helpful to know the gene defect, i.e. the sequence of the corresponding gene. For this purpose the DNA-carrying the gene has to be identified and isolated. Genes such as the insulin gene can be found using the fact that its corresponding mRNA is enriched in specific tissue. For about 500 disease-related genes, however, only their approximate position on one of the chromosomes is known.

There is a wide variety of strategies to find out which chromosome or chromosome band defects are correlated with a certain disease. In a few cases, however, the matter is surprisingly simple. For example, when primarily boys, suffer from a disease or abnormality (some muscular diseases, bleeding disease, several types of color blindness) then one concludes that the correlated gene must be located on the X chromosome of which boys have only one whereas girls have a "spare" chromosome which may compensate the defect. (The Y chromosome may also be involved, but due to its small size the probability is low.) When, in addition, a look into the microscope reveals that there is a morphological anomaly on the X-chromosome, then even the chromosomal region is known, where one gene or a group of genes contributing to the disease may be located. This is the case in fragile X disease in chromosomal region Xq27-28, which causes metal retardation. Presently this obviously important region of the human genome is being systematically sequenced.

Localizing the position of a disease gene on one of the autosomes is not as simple as for the sex related genetic diseases. Occasionally one finds that the order of genes or other sequences in the genome of a person carrying the disease has been consistently rearranged. Even if the rearranged sequence is not involved in the disease itself, it can serve as a marker. When in 100 persons carrying a given disease one has a rearranged marker sequence the distance of the marker to the putative disease gene is defined as

1 centimorgan.

In other words the centimorgan is a genetic distance between two positions in a genome expressed as a percentage of rearranged events. As a rule of thumb, in human DNA one centimorgan corresponds to one megabase, but there are recombinational hotspots in the human genome where this estimate may be completely wrong.

When a marker sequence is found which is almost always rearranged in persons carrying a disease, one knows that the unknown gene must be very close. Unfortunately establishing this is a tedious task and may take decades. Microdissection and microcloning (see Section 5.4) may help to speed up this process. Finding the position of a disease gene in a genome has been termed "positional cloning". The disease genes for cystic fibrosis and for Huntington's disease have been found via this technique. In Box 69 the frequency of selected inheritable diseases in the European and North American populations is given.

**Box 69: Frequency of selected genetic diseases**

| | |
|---|---|
| Duchenne and Becker Dystrophy | 1/4000 |
| Hemophilia A | 1/8000 |
| Hemophilia B | 1/30000 |
| Mental retardation with fragile X chromosome | 1/1500 |
| Other X-linked mental diseases | 1/1000 |

However, these frequencies vary significantly in different populations. This is shown in Box 70 for the frequency of cystic fibrosis in the Mediterranean region, where people of different genetic origin live under similar environmental circumstances.

**Box 70: Cystic fibrosis in different Mediterranean populations:**
**Ratio of disease carriers to all others**

| | |
|---|---|
| Ashkenazi | 1:3300 |
| Lybians | 1:2700 |
| Georgians | 1:2700 |
| Greek/Bulkgarian | 1:2400 |
| Yemenites | 1:8800 |
| Marrocans | 1:15000 |
| Iraqui | 1:32000 |
| Irani | 1:39000 |

This box shows that, even if a disease is presumed to be caused primarily by one single gene, this does not solely regulate the frequency of the disease.

Other genes are associated with increased risk of cancer. Cancer related genes may be either deleted or amplified, mutated or under- or overexpressed. It is quite difficult to say if the modification of a given gene is a cause or a consequence of cancer. Box 71 gives a list of such genes.

**Box 71: Cloned genes associated with increased risk of cancer (From Nelson, 1996)**

| Gene | Chromosome | Cancer predisposition |
|------|-----------|----------------------|
| p53 | 17p13.1 | Breast cancer, soft tissue sarcomas, bone cancer, brain tumors leukemia, adrenocortical carcinoma |
| RB1 | 13q14.3 | Childhood tumors of the eye (retinoblastoma) |
| WT1 | 11p13 | Childhood kidney tumors (Wilms tumor) |
| NF1 | 17q11.2 | Nerve tumors (neurofibromatosis) |
| NF2 | 22q12.2 | Acoustic nerve and brain tumors (neurofibromatosis) |
| VHL | 3p25 | Benign and malignant tumors in kidney, retina, central nervous system, pancreas, adrenal glands (von Hippel Lindau disease) |
| MTS1 or p16 | 9p21 | Malignant melanoma, pancreatic cancer |
| RET | 19q11.2 | Multiple endocrine neoplasias, thyroid and adrenal cancer |
| MSH 2 | 2p16 | Colorectal cancer |
| MLH 1 | 3p21 | Colorectal cancer, hereditary non-polyposis colon cancer (HNPCC) |
| BRCA 1 | 17q21 | Breast cancer |
| BRCA 2 | 13q12 | Breast and ovarian cancer |
| CDK 4 | | Melanoma |

## Selected literature

F.C. Collins (1995) Ahead schedule and under budget: The genome project passes its fifth birthday. Proc. Natl. Acad. Sci. 92, 10821–23.

N.J. Nelson (1996) Cloned genes associated with cancer risk. J. Natl. Cancer Institute 88, 72.

T.J. Hudson et al. (1995) An STS based map of the human genome. Science 270, 1945–1954.

# 5.4 Laser microdissection of chromosomes

You know either from the previous chapter or from your education in biology that genomes consist of several thousands to ten thousands of genes and that in the human genome the localization of many of them in specific chromosome bands is known. About 600 chromosomal positions can now be correlated with human diseases as a result of extended cytogentic studies. The molecular basis of about additional 4000 human diseases is suspected to have their origin in the DNA. Only for a few of them are the molecular details already known, i.e. the disease can already be correlated with the DNA sequence.

## 5.4.1 The motivation for microdissection of chromosomes

In the present chapter, laser microdissection and subsequent microcloning of metaphase chromosomes will be described. A chromosome segment obtained by laser microdissection is used to clone the DNA contained in it. The result will be a set (a library) of DNA probes specific for the given chromosome segment.

It is highly tedious and may take years to achieve a precise localization and, finally, identification of the gene correlated to the disease. One example is the gene for cystic fibrosis, which for several years was known to be located on the human chromosome 7, band q22-q32. Using this knowledge, molecular geneticists were able to isolate DNA from this chromosomal region and finally identify one DNA clone which contained the gene. After sequencing this DNA it was quickly found that a defect in a transmembrane channel, the cystic fibrosis transmembrane receptor CFTR, is involved in causing the disease. This knowledge may be useful for those who develop therapies against this fatal disease and may finally significantly contribute to defeating it. For Huntington's disease, for example, even 15 years of intensive research have brought success only after stretches of chromosomes were systematically sequenced. And another 600 diseases are awaiting analysis.

One reason for the slow progress may be the fact that usually the whole genome has to be investigated. Isolation of a narrow region around the disease locus on a chromosome by dissecting chromosome in metaphase preparations in a suitable way may help to speed up that process. Thus, microdissection is gaining importance in cytogenetics and molecular genetics.

## 5.4.2 Microdissection of chromosomes

Mechanical microdissection of chromosomes is possible but requires a skilled experimentator. Laser microdissection, in contrast, is simple. Once a laser microbeam is set up, it is easy to learn and perform microdissection of chromosomes. (Monajembashi et al., 1986). Fig. 30 (from Eckelt et al., 1989) shows how the largest chromosome isolated from a human metaphase is microdissected with the laser microbeam.

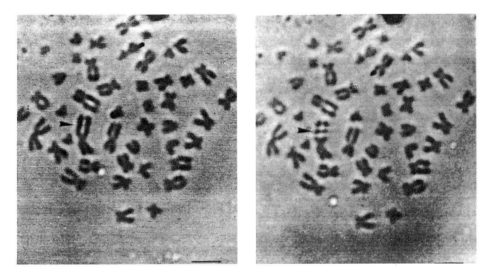

**Fig. 30:** Top: A preparation of the chromosomes from a human blood cell. The donor of the cell has a translocation (combination) between chromosomes #1 and #7, which is the largest chromosome in the preparation. Bottom: The translocation chromosome is microdissected at the fusion site of the two chromosomes.

Human chromosomes have a length of a few micrometers and can, alternatively to laser mirodissection, also be dissected micromechanically. Mechanical microdissection of the small chromosomes of some plants such as the rapeseed *Brassica napus* is not practical. These chromosomes are very small and quite often appear only as dots in a normal microscope. In synchronized fixed cells of *Brassica napus* chromosomes were microdissected at 4000x magnification (Fig. 31).

With laser microdissection, a large area around the microdisected chromosome segment can be ablated so that the latter lies comparably free on the coverslide. Several approaches are available to pick up the chromosome segment. One way would

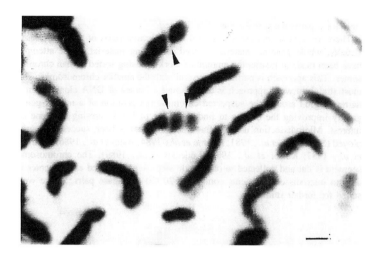

**Fig. 31:** *Laser microdissection of rapeseed chromosomes.*

be to use a microneedle. At first glance this does not appear to be very clever: if a microneedle has to be used anyway, one can also perform the microdissection with the needle. However, combined microdissection and microhandling with the needle requires micrometer accuracy. When microdissection is performed by the laser microbeam, the chromosome segment can be prepared with a free space of 10 micrometers around it and thus microhandling can be performed with a lower accuracy, say 10 micrometers. A second experimental strategy is to remove all of the unwanted chromosomal material and to rinse the desired chromosome segments from the microscope slide. (Djabali, 1991). Finally the chromosome slice can be transported by optical tweezers (see below).

When a chromosome with more complex geometry has to be dissected, laser microdissection is often the only method available. At sufficiently high laser power (with an excimer laser pumped dye laser) one can use the system of diffraction rings instead of the central Airy disk (see Appendix A3) to make almost equidistant cuts in a chromosome. Since the ring thickness is given by the wavelength, one can vary it easily just by changing the wavelength of the dye laser. A second type of cut is particularly simple to perform with laser microdissection if one is interested in DNA material which is located in the flanks of a chromosome. The cut can be set along, instead across, the chromosomes and thus can separate the two chromatids and delete material either close to the long chromosome axis or, alternatively, at the flanks. Fig. 32 shows one of these geometries.

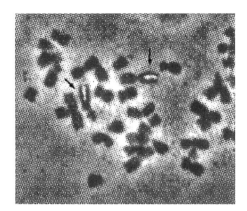

**Fig. 32:** *Chromosome cut along the long axis in order to separate the two chromatids (From Monajembashi et al., 1997).*

## 5.4.3 Submicroscopic effects of laser microdissection

Having in mind the experiments where chromosomes were severed rather than really cut (Section 3.1) it is difficult to believe that laser microdissection is an adequate tool for preparing chromosome segment-specific DNA probes. However, in the microsevering experiments lasers of moderate intensity (power density) or lasers working in the visible had been used. Near diffraction limited pulsed UV lasers, such as the nitrogen laser, make a difference. This has been discussed in Section 2.2.3, where it was shown that the laser ablates exactly where it hits a sample but causes only minor change to the immediate surroundings. An electron microscopic study shows that with unstained chromosomes, a nitrogen-laser microbeam works with good accuracy in the submicrometer range (Ponelies et al., 1989).

One can see that the cut is clear, the edges are sharp. Occasionally one observes that the laser produces a hole in the supporting microscope glass when it hits directly while no such defects are seen under the cut, i.e. where the glass was protected by the chromosome. This is an example of the precision which can be obtained with a pulsed UV laser microbeam. For the human chromosome band 9q34, the group of Berns (He et al.,1997) has compared laser microdissection with micromechanical dissection and came also to the conclusion, that higher precision at comparable quality of the results can be obtained.

Laser microdissection can also be combined with microdissection by the tip of an atomic force microscope. Alternatively the chromosome is dissected with the laser microbeam and the result is directly observed with the AFM (Thalhammer et al., 1997). These experiments also reveal minimal damage caused by UV laser microbeams.

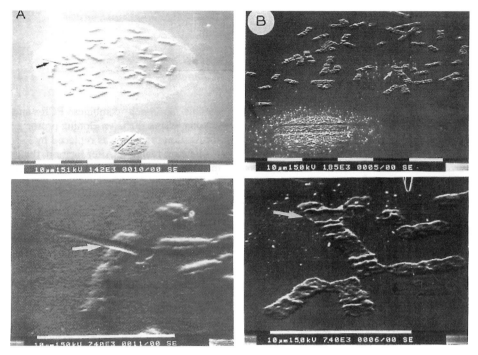

*Fig. 33:* Electron micrographs of laser dissected Drosophila chromosomes from different angles.

## 5.4.4 Combined use of laser microbeam and optical tweezers

In spite of the fact that one single chromosome segment is sufficient to allow for a few DNA probes, there are experiments where it is desirable to have a large number of segments. The combination of laser microbeam and optical tweezers permits the isolation of a large number of such chromosome segments: Fig. 34 shows schematically how a chromosome can first be cut with the microbeam and then be transported with the trap.

In Fig. 35 it is shown how laser microbeam and optical tweezers are used in combination for microdissection of the tip of a chromosome in suspension and for the subsequent isolation of the dissected segment without mechanical contact.

This approach allows one to prepare hundreds of segments from chromosomes in suspension within a few hours. Since this process can be semi-automated, it is conceivable that a thousand or more chromosome segments per day can be prepared. A present drawback of the technique is the need for unstained chromosomes in suspension, a requirement which reduces the spatial accuracy of the microdissection. This problem may, however, be solved by finding a compromise between

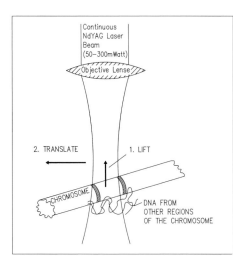

**Fig. 34:** *Schematic representation of the combined use of laser microbeam and optical tweezers to isolate chromosome segments.*

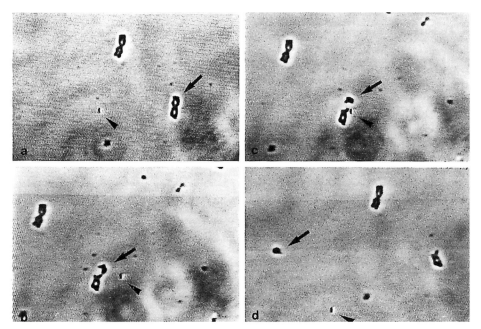

**Fig. 35:** *Cutting and transport of a chromosome segment. The large arrow marks the chromosome segment, the small arrow the position of the optical trap.*

experimental conditions where non-fixed chromosomes in suspension and metaphase preparations adhering strongly to the microscope slide are used. Thus the microbeam and optical tweezers may become a suitable tool for rapid and convenient isolation of chromosome segments.

195

## 5.4.5 Microcloning

The chromosome segments obtained by microdissection represent, in principle, highly condensed chromatin (see Sections 5.3.1 and 5.3.2). Their protein content has to be digested away, often using the enzyme proteinase K. This and all subsequent steps have to be performed in microdroplets or in microvessels. After protein digestion the DNA has to be amplified.

Techniques available for amplification of DNA include cloning into phages, cloning into plasmids or cosmids, and several PCR based techniques (degenerate oligonucleotide primer PCR; adapter PCR; IRS, PCR, particularly Alu-PCR) (see Box 72).

The first laser microdissection experiments used microcloning into lambda phage for the generation of DNA probes (Eckelt et al., 1989, Ponelies et al., 1989). Picograms of DNA in nanoliter volumes are available as starting material. From about 100 human metaphases, chromosome segments from region 7q22–q32 were isolated, collectively digested by the restriction endonuclease EcoR1 and cloned into the lambda bacteriophage vector NM 1149. This vector was then amplified in the selective *E. coli* strain NM 514. Fourhundred and fifty clones were obtained, 220 of them were of low copy number. Twenty clones were analyzed by gel electrophoresis and had an average size of 3.8 kb. Four clones were tested by in situ hybridization, three of them could be localized in bands 7q22-32. Fig. 36 shows an electrophoresis gel on which selected clones from this library were characterized according to their size.

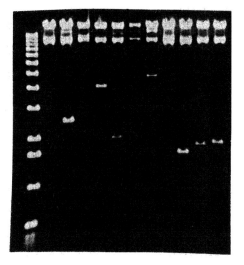

**Fig. 36:** *Gel electrophoretic characterization of DNA clones obtained by laser microdissection and microcloning into lambda phage. Seven clones are tested. They all have different sizes as can be seen by comparison with the size marker (the ladder on the left). Thus one can infer that the clones are all different.*

## Box 72: Cloning into phages and into cosmids

The basic strategy of phage cloning is to insert (ligate) the piece of DNA to be amplified into host DNA which is amplified by a natural process. Viruses (coli bacteriophages such as the bacteriophages fd, M13 or the lambda phage) which specifically infect *Escherichia coli* have been found to be suitable. They are safe in the sense that they do not infect human cells or cells from other higher organisms.

In order to insert foreign DNA into the DNA of lambda phage one has to find a restriction endonuclease which can cut the natural phage DNA at a suitable site. The foreign DNA is then trimmed by the same endonuclease (quite often a special trimming step is not really necessary since "digests" from large DNA using the same endonuclease are used anyway. Since both, foreign DNA and phage DNA, now have the same cutting ends, they fit each other and a ligase can combine them into one single recombined DNA molecules. In one strategy, they are mixed with coat proteins of lambda phage. These proteins and the DNA assemble without outer help into new, infectious lambda phages. When they are mixed with E. coli bacteria they infect them and multiply as most other viruses multiply, thereby amplifying the foreign DNA molecules. Finally, the phage DNA is isolated and purified and the desired piece of DNA is cut out from the phage DNA by the same endonucleases which were previously used for trimming.

Without any precautions phages containing the desired DNA and native phages grow equally well and in the end one has difficulties in distinguishing them. Therefore, modified lambda phages are used which contain part of a gene coding for a colored material. Exactly in this gene there is the cutting site for the trimming endonuclease, i.e. foreign DNA will finally be inserted exactly into this site, thereby disrupting the color gene. Thus, when a phage without foreign DNA infects *E. coli*, the colony (clone) will be blue. Phages with inserts, i.e. with disrupted color gene, will result in white colonies. Thus it is easy to single out those colonies which contain foreign DNA by selecting the white colonies.

The whole cloning process is somewhat tedious but has the advantage that foreign DNA up to 20 kilobases can be inserted into the DNA of lambda phages. Special constructs, the cosmids, take up to 45 kilobases. A third group of vectors, as these carriers of foreign DNA are called, are the yeast artificial chromosomes (YACs, not to confuse with YAG which is laser medium) . They can take up to 1 megabase of DNA, but are difficult to handle. These are extrachromosomal ring-like DNA elements which directly, i.e without their being packed into protein envelopes, can infect certain bacteria. They usually accept up to 10 kilobases and are more flexible than phage DNA with respect to artificially introduced restriction sites and markers for inserted DNA.

## 5.4.6 PCR (Polymerase Chain Reaction)
(for detailed information see, for example, K. Mullis, 1994)

Cloning into lambda phages requires 10 to 100 chromosome segments. PCR techniques are more sensitive and yield results already with a single chromosome segment.

Due to its sensitivity, PCR is increasingly replacing phage microcloning (see for example Lüdecke 1989, Melzer el al., 1992). PCR, as a pure enzyme reaction, requires no safety measures. A disadvantage is that the amplified DNA pieces are usually shorter than those obtained by the phage cloning.

Conceptually, the PCR is simple. To some extent it imitates transcription. Single-stranded DNA molecules are used as a template and a DNA polymerase synthesizes a complementary strand. DNA polymerase needs a double-stranded starting site. This is generated by hybridizing short single-stranded "primer" to the target molecule. Primers are single stranded oligonucleotides, 15–30 bases in length, which are complemetary to sequence elements of the DNA to be amplified. When the primer sequence is known exactly it can be hybridized to the single-stranded DNA molecule under very stringent conditions, i.e. in a very exact way. Such ideal primers can be used to amplify a piece of DNA contained in a large mixture of unwanted DNA molecules. In fact, it can find "the needle in the haystack".

Often the thermostable Taq (thermus aquaticus) polymerase is used. DNA amplification can then be performed in a single vessel experiment.

After mixing the components (DNA template, the primers, the polymerase and nucleotides) the temperature is regulated in a well-defined manner between low (<40 °C, where DNA exists as a double-strand) and high temperatures (above 80 °C where the DNA melts into single strands). For temperature-dependent DNA melting, see Box 75). Typically 30 of such cycles are employed, each taking approximately three minutes. The thermal cycling allows one to separate the whole reaction into three phases (for details see Box 73).

In each cycle the number of DNA molecules is doubled. After 20 cycles the amplification factor is 1 million; then the number of DNA molecules thereafter ceases to grow exponentially due to primer and nucleotide consumption and due to amplification errors.

When unknown DNA has to be amplified as it is the case in laser microdissection experiments the primer binding site is not known, i.e. an exact primer to start the polymerase chain reaction cannot be constructed. There are, howevever, several possibilities to use intrinsic sequence elements as primer binding sites. These are summarized in Box 74.

As already shown for Alu-PCR, PCR-mediated approaches work with extremely low amounts of DNA. The vector-PCR and adaptor-PCR are combined with modified microcloning, in which the ligation reaction between adaptor and foreign DNA seems to be more efficient than the ligation of plasmid with foreign DNA. SUP-PCR (single unique primer-PCR) as well as the Alu-PCR do not require microcloning.

### Box 73: Steps of PCR

#### Denaturation

At high temperature: Double strands, synthesized in a previous cycle are separated into two single strands. Each of them may serve as a template for the next amplification step.

#### Primer annealing

At low temperature: Here the primers bind to the sequence elements to which they are complementary.

#### Elongation

At intermediate temperature: Now the polymerases can work and synthesize the strand complementarily to the respective template.

In laser microbeam experiments, PCR has, for example, been employed to amplify segments from region Xq27.3, which is the locus for the fragile X syndrome (Hadano, 1991). There, either the repetitive Alu sequences of the human genome or known sequences of vectors into which the DNA was ligated, have been used as PCR primers. Up to $2 \cdot 10^4$ clones with insert sizes of a factor of 10 smaller than those frm lambda cloning were obtained. They were used to characterize a library of segment-specific cosmids organized as a matrix on a substrate (a gridded library). Eight clones out of 384 were recognized by the laser dissected clones.

For the human chromosome band 4q35, a laser microdissection library has been constructed with the aim to fine-map the region responsible for facio-capulohumoral muscular dystrophy (Uphadya et al., 1995). This disease is characterized by weakness of muscles in the face and the shoulder. For the experiment a sophisticated chromosome microdissector based on an argon ion laser was used. This is a combination of a laser microbeam with an imaging processing system which allows automatic preparation of single chromosome segments. From the dissection of one metaphase, a very large number of clones with an average insert size of 340 bp were obtained. When a sample of 70 clones was sequenced it turned out that only 57 were different, i.e. 13 clone pairs were at least doubled. In such a case one has to carefully consider the statistics of the sample: this result may mean that "the contents" of the library is quite redundant, i.e. that many clones are identical. Nevertheless, at least 50 clones are different from each other and this means a clone density hardly obtainable by any other method.

Laser microdissection has also been used to construct libraries from plant chromosomes (Fukui et al., 1992; Ponelies et al., 1997) and has thus shown the broad range of applicability of laser microdissection.

## Summary and outlook

By laser microdissection of metaphase chromosomes one can gain access to stretches of DNA which are related to a specific phenotype or to a specific disease. Microdissected chromosome segments can be isolated by transporting the microdissected chromosome segments to a preselected position on the microscope slide.

### Box 74: Different variants of PCR

#### Adaptor-PCR

This approach combines PCR and microcloning. Using the microcloning protocol, the vector-ligation reaction was replaced by linker-adaptor-ligation reaction. After ligation, the nanoliter-mixture is transferred into a PCR-reaction tube where the amplification takes place with use of one adaptor-oligonucleotide as primer. Finally the PCR product is digested with the defined restriction enzyme and cloned into a vector. Thus microamplification of the chromosomal starting material facilitates the reduction of the number of needed chromosome segments.

#### DOP-PCR

(Degenerate oligonucleotide primer PCR). This is one representative of a whole class of PCR techniques where a primer fits only very approximately a target sequence is used. In order to allow binding in spite of the fact that the primer does not really fit, the "stringency" of the primer binding has to be reduced by decreasing the temperature (for the temperature effects see Table 6) of the annealing process or by adding suitable chemicals. Many variants of this strategy exist.

## ALU-PCR

*Alu*-PCR uses repetitive sequences in the human genome ($3.10^5$–$9.10^5$ Alu-sequences per haploid human genome), with an average distance of about 4-5 kb as primer. They are enriched in the dark Giemsa bands of chromosomes (R-bands). More than a third of the *Alu*-sequences is separated by less than 1 kb single copy DNA (and can be used as primer binding sites. With standard protocols the DNA of a few hundred segments (ca. 30 fg each) would be required for *Alu*-PCR.With higher concentrations of $MgCl_2$, primer and nucleotides (12 mM MgCl2, 1.8 µM primer and 1 mM each nucleotide) and $^5$TGC ACT CCA GCC TGG G$^3$ corresponding to the $^3$-end of an Alu-consensus sequence as primer and treatment with DNase I (Boehringer Mannheim, Germany, 5 units, 45 min, 37 °C) to avoid amplification of contaminating DNA, single molecule sensitivity can be obtained .

## Box 75: Melting temperatures for oligonucleotides of different composition and different length

In PCR, double strands have to be denatured into single strands. Upon increasing the temperature, the DNA gradually melts. The midpoint of this process, which covers many centigrades is defined as the melting temperature. It is possible to estimate the melting temperature from the content of guanine and cytosine in the DNA, the G+C content. A number of different empirical formula exist. For nucleotides up to 30 base pairs in length

$$Tm = 4 (G+C) + 2 (A+T)$$

yields reasonable values for the melting temperature. The table below gives some melting temperatures for different short DNA molecules

| length | G+C | A+T | $T_m$ (°C) |
|--------|-----|-----|------------|
| 10 | 0 | 10 | 20 |
| 10 | 5 | 5 | 30 |
| 10 | 10 | 0 | 40 |
| 20 | 20 | 0 | 80 |

For long DNA molecules often the following formula is used

$$T_m = -16.6 \log [S] + 41.5 X_{GC} + 81.5 \quad (38)$$

where $T_m$ is the melting temperature in degrees centigrade, [S] is the concentration of monovalent salt ions in mol per liter and $X_{GC}$ is the mol fraction (percentage divided by 100) of G and C bases. At low salt concentrations, the melting temperature often is calculated to be above 100 °C.

## Selected literature

M. Djabali, C. Nguyen, I. Biunno, B.A. Oostra, M.G. Mattei, J.E. Ikeda and B.R. Jordan (1991) Laser microdissection of the fragile X region: identification of cosmid clones and of conserved sequences in this region. Genomics 10: 1053–1060.

A. Eckelt, N. Ponelies, E.K.F. Bautz, K. Miller, T. Heuer, B. Tümmler, K.H. Grzeschik, J. Wolfrum and K.O. Greulich (1989) Microdissection in the search for the molecular basis of disease: A chromosome segment specific molecular library. Ber. Bunsenges. Phys. Chem. 93, 1446.

S. Fukui et al. (1992) Microdissection of plant chromosomes by an argon ion laser beam. Theor. Appl. Genetics 84.7–8, 787–794.

S. Hadano, M. Watanabe, H. Yokiu, M. Kogi, I. Kondo, H. Tsuchiya, I. Kanazawa, K. Wakasa, J. Ikeda (1991) Laser microdissection and single unique primer PCR allow generation of regional chromosome DNA clones from a single human chromosome. Genomics 11, 364–373.

W. He, Y. Liu, M. Smith and M.W. Berns (1997) Laser microdissection for gnereation of a human chromosome region specific library. Microsc. Microanal. 3, 47–52.

H.J. Lüdecke, G. Senger, U. Claussen and B. Horsthemke (1989) Cloning defined regions of the human genome by microdissection of banded chromosomes and enzymatic amplification. Nature 338, 348–350.

P.S. Melzer, X.Y. Guan, A. Burgess and J.M. Trent (1992) Rapid generation of region specific probes by chromosome microdissection and their application. Nature Genetics 1, 24-28.

S. Monajembashi, C. Cremer, T. Cremer, J. Wolfrum and K.O. Greulich (1986) Microdissection of chromosomes by a laser microbeam. Exp. Cell Research 167, 262.

S. Monajembashi, C. Hoyer and K.O. Greulich (1997) Laser Microbeams and optical tweezers convert the microscope into a versatile microtool. Microscopy and Analysis, 97.1, 7–9.

K.B. Mullis, F. Ferre and R.A. Gibbs (1994) The Polymerase chain Reaction. Birkhäuser, Boston.

N. Ponelies, E.K.F. Bautz, S. Monajembashi, J. Wolfrum and K.O. Greulich (1989)

Telomeric sequences derived from laser-microdissected polytene chromosomes. Chromosoma 98, 351–357.

N. Ponelies, N. Stein and G. Weber (1997) Microamplification of specific chromosome sequences; an improved method for genome analysis. Nucl. Acids. Res. 25, 3555–3557.

S. Thalhammer, R.W. Stark, K. Schütze, J. Wienberg and W.M. Heckl (1997) Laser microdissection of metaphase chromosomes and characterization by atomic force microscopy. J. Biom. Optics 2 (1), 115–119.

M. Upadhyaya, M. Osborn, J. Maynard, M. Altherr, J. Ikeda and P.S. Harper (1995) Towards the finer mapping of faciocapulohumoral muscular dystrophy at 4q35: construction of a laser microdissection library. J. Med. Gen. 60, 244–251.

# 6 From biology to medicine

Knowing how an organism develops from an egg, learning details about cell division, manipulating molecular motors – nice, but basic research! But aren there even more practical applications? Indeed there are!

The last part of our journey through the world of applications will lead us to techniques as different as laser-assisted gene transfer, cell fusion, measurements of properties of blood cells, immunology and, finally, to the use of laser microtools in *in vitro* fertilization. Among these techniques are a few which may in the not too far future find their use in plant breeding, medical diagnostics or therapy and in cancer research.

## 6.1 Laser microtools in plant cell biology

Many plant cells are transparent, and one can easily recognize intracellular details. Such cells are particularly suitable to demonstrate the power of laser microtools, particularly their suitability to work in the interior of closed objects.

### 6.1.1 Optical trapping in the interior of plant cells

In order to get access to intracellular structures, for microinjection as well as for basic research, it is desirable to have control over the position of subcellular structures such as mitochondria and chloroplasts. An early study on internal cell manipulation in rapeseed cells has shown that in this cell type subcellular organelles are particular mobile. They can be pulled through the cell with high spatial control. Fig. 37, taken from Greulich et al., 1989, shows the result.

The alga *Pyrocystis noctiluca* is ideally suited for demonstrating the potential of laser microtechniques as an intracellular working tool. It is transparent at almost all optical wavelengths and structures inside the cell are well visible. The cell has a type of skeleton made of cytoplasmic strands which stabilize the overall structure. Major parts of the cells appear to be empty. This is the vacuole, surrounded by a membrane, the tonoplast.

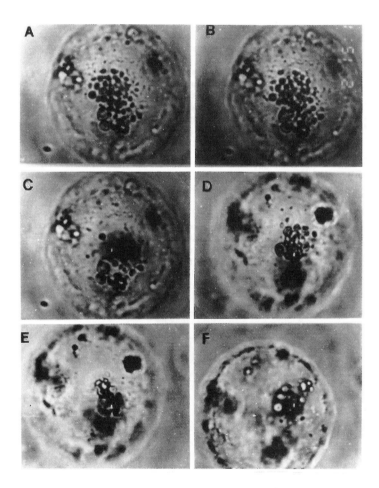

**Fig. 37:** *Moving subcellular structures in the interior of rapeseed cells. A to C shows a preselected object plane in the microscope. The focus of the optical trap is not exactly in the object plane but somewhat behind it. When the trap is switched on, the subcellular particles disappear below the object plane. After refocusing one can find them again, now clustered in the focus of the trapping laser. D. Moving the latter (E and F) allows one to move the particles to almost any position in the cell.*

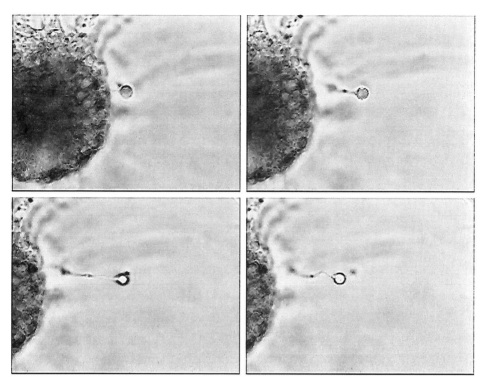

**Fig. 38:** *Displacement (top) of an organelle by optical tweezers in the interior of an unopened cell of Pyrocystis noctiluca and subsequent return movement (bottom).*

Two types of laser micromanipulation experiments can be performed (Leitz et al., 1994): By microdissection of the cytoplasmic strands one can test how many of them are really required for maintaining the cell's integrity, see Fig. 21 on page 118. With optical tweezers it is possible to displace subcellular organelles and thereby obtain information on the compartmentation of the cell and on intracellular viscosities.

In the second type of experiment single chloroplasts were displaced with optical tweezers (laser power at microscope entrance 700 mW). In most routine experiments the organelles are displaced over a distance of 50 mm. After release they migrated back at variable speeds, Fig. 38 shows this process.

One can clearly recognize that the organelle remains connected to its original position by a membrane filament, probably part of the tonoplast membrane and that it is this connection which finally drives the organelle back to its original position. Depending on the absolute distance of elongation this may occur almost elastically. In the sequence of events shown here the elongation was too large and some plastic deformation of the membrane filament can be seen. Generally, immediately after the optical tweezers are switched off, the organelle begins to retreat at high speed; this speed gradually decreases as the organelle approaches its original position. Box 76 lists the speed of return after trapping over different duration at a distance of 20 μm.

**Box 76: Speed of organelle return movement after different trapping times in *Pyrocystis noctiluca***

| Duration of trapping | Speed of movement (μm/s) |
| --- | --- |
| 0 min | 81.7 ± 7.8 |
| 1 min | 4.2 ± 0.2 |
| 5 min | 2.6 ± 0.3 |
| 15 min | 1.8 ± 0.2 |

All speeds were determined on the basis of 10 experiments except the value at 0 min which was based on 25 different cells. It is obvious that at an elongation of 20 μm for 1 min or more causes inelastic weakening of the membrane filament.

The return movement is also temperature dependent. For these measurement the cells were kept at a given temperature for a few minutes. i.e. temperature equilibrium can be assumed. Box 77 presents the results.

**Box 77: Initial speed for return movement at different temperatures**

| Temperature | Speed (μm/s) |
| --- | --- |
| 2 °C | 34.5.± 2.7 |
| 25 °C | 81.7 ± 7.8 |
| 30 °C | 94.5 ± 9.0 |

The increase of speed with temperature can be explained by a decreased intracellular viscosity at increased temperatures. In a crude approximation the initial speed depends linearly on temperature. Thus it may, in turn, be used to aquire a first idea about thermal effects caused by the NdYAG laser.

## 6.1.2 Simulating microgravity in the alga *Chara*

The alga *Chara* has specific tube like cells, the rhizoids, which it uses to sense gravity. Under normal conditions the rhizoids always grow downward, i.e. toward the direction of higher gravity. While the detailed mechanism for this "gravitropism" is not understood, some facts are known: Close to the tips of the rhizoids dense structures, 1–2 µm in diameter, can be recognized. These structures, called statoliths, are barium sulfate microcrystals enveloped by membranes. Obviously they sediment under the influence of gravity and control the direction of growth.

They have a higher refractive index than the environment and thus can easily be caught and moved by optical tweezers in the interior of living rhizoids. (Leitz et al., 1995). It is not only possible to move one statolith but up to 5 of such structures can be collected in the focus of the optical tweezers and held permanently. The force required for displacement depends on the direction of displacement, i.e. if it occurs in the direction of the main cell body (basipetal), in the opposite direction (acropetal) or perpendicularly to the axis of the tube like rhizoid (lateral). Box 78 lists the laser power, i.e. an uncalibrated measure of the actual force, required to move the statoliths in a different direction. Also, in order to get some idea about the underlying mechanism, the outcome of the experiments in the presence of cytochalasin B (cyt B) is included.

**Box 78: Laser power (in mW) required to move statoliths in a different direction**

|  | Without cyt B | With cyt B |
|---|---|---|
| Lateral (perpendicular to tube axis) | 210 | 200 |
| Acropetal (towards tip) | 350 | 210 |
| Basipetal (away from tip) | 480 | 250 |

These data give some information on the role of actin in holding the statoliths in place. Cyt B is known to destabilize actin. Actin induces a vigorous movement of subcellular particles in the direction of the tip and back, but not so much perpendicular to the long axis of the rhizoid. In other words, there are active forces in the direction of the long axis and it is difficult to hold streaming particles, on the one hand, or to move fixed particles on the other hand, against these forces. When cyt B disrupts the actin, those forces are no longer present. The laser power required to work against these forces is then reduced. In the lateral direction there is obviously no stabilizing force provided by actin.

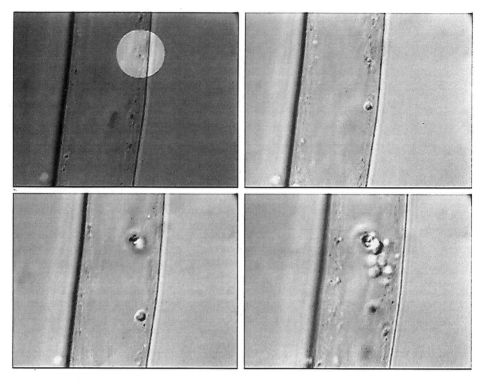

**Fig. 39:** *Particles in a cytoplasmic stream stopped by optical tweezers. Only in the bottom right figure can a major group of particles be seen in the vigorous stream of other particles.*

Apart from the statoliths, a large variety of subcellular particles are transported in the rhizoid by a vigorous streaming with approximately 3 µm/s. Selected particles can be stopped from outside the cell and held by the optical tweezers, for example, for inspection or for an indirect measurement of their refractive index. Fig. 39 shows such a group of particles held with the tweezers. In this still micrograph the background is blurred due to the vigorous motion of all other particles not held by the tweezers. How does displacement of statoliths influence growth of the rhizoids? So far, experiments to tackle this problem had to be performed either in the Earth's orbit or microgravity had to be simulated a slow rotating centrifuge microscope. For a short time, microgravity towers or parabolic flights of aircrafts or rockets could also simulate space conditions to some extent. Experiments using optical tweezers are much simpler to perform, can extend for hours and do not perturb other elements of a cell. In such experiments, statoliths are displaced from their original exposition as described above and growth is observed, typically by video recording. Fig. 40 (from Leitz et al., 1995) shows a *Chara* rhizoid at different times.

The figure shows the microcrystals in the tip region of the alga and it shows the deviation of growth induced by the optical trap. Control experiments illuminating the same region but not removing the crystals do not change the growth direction, i.e., in the present experiment growth is not just affected by a thermal effect. At time zero the statoliths are in their original position, determined by gravity. At all other times, up to more than three hours, the statoliths are displaced. The rhizoids no longer grow towards gravity. That is approximately what one had expected. In other words, the hypothesis that the statoliths mediate gravity-sensing is correct. More surprising is the fact that not only the direction, but also the speed of growth is changed, and that this effect makes almost an order of magnitude. Fig. 41 shows in the upper part, the apical displacement of the statoliths. The lower part, on the same

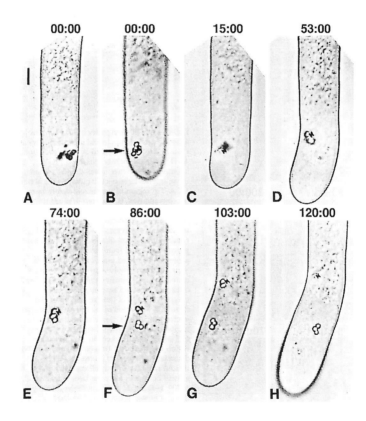

**Fig. 40:** Micrographs of one Chara rhizoid after different durations of statolith displacement. The micrographs are mounted together to give an impression on the temporal course. The times at the top of each partial figure are given in minutes.

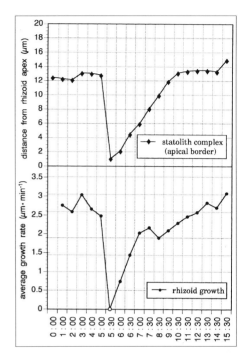

**Fig. 41:** *Upper part: Distance of the statolith complex in Chara from the tip of the rhizoid. The distance under normal gravitation is approx. 13 μm. The rhizoid is allowed to grow normally for the first 5 min of the experiment. Then, the statolith complex is displaced. Immediately the growth rate (lower part of the figure) decreases from 2.8 μm/sec to almost zero and recovers as the statolith complex returns to its original position. Statolith position and tip growth rate. (From: Leitz et al., 1995.)*

time scale gives the growth rate of the tip. Note that in this representation the relaxed position of the statoliths is at approximately 13 μm.

One can see that statolith displacement and tip growth are highly correlated. At most, there is a slight delay of the growth rate. These results provoke some speculation. May it be that evolution has optimized tip growth for Earth's gravitational acceleration and that a deviation from this results in suboptimal growth rates? An answer can only be given when other plants have been investigated in similar ways.

## 6.1.3 Preparing free plant membranes for patch clamp studies

Laser microsurgery has a completely different aim when it is applied with view to combining it with plant electrophysiology. In such cases, one would like to record the electrical activity of individual channel molecules in the cell membrane by measuring the picoampere currents of membrane patches electrically sealed with a very fine micropipette (patch clamping). Patch clamping has been widely used in animal cell membrane research. Plant cells, however, have a hard cell wall in addition to the more fatty cell membrane. Often, in order to get access to the membrane, the cell wall is removed by digestion of the wall with an enzyme cocktail, i.e one prepares wall-free protoplasts enzymatically. The disadvantage of this process is that the membrane properties are changed and the patch clamping results may not reflect the *in vivo* situation.

For some plants the laser can provide access to much more native membrane: when, for example, the root hairs of *Medigaco sativae* are cut at their tip (Kurkdjian et al., 1993), internal pressure expells the protoplast. Fig. 42 shows that process.

By staining with the dye Tinopal (alternatively with "Calcofluore white") which would cause a blue fluorescence if cell wall components were still present it can be shown that pure membrane is prepared. For the first 10 minutes after microsurgery no staining is observed, i.e. within that time frame one has access to a true plant cell membrane.

De Boer et al. (1994) have extended these studies and shown for four further types of plants that access to membranes can be gained by laser microsurgery. In total the following cell types were studied:

1  tobacco (*Nicotiana tabacum*)
2  an unicellular green alga (*Eremosphera viridis*)
3  an angiospermic plant (*Elodes densa*)
4  lili pollen tubes (*Lilium longiflorum*).

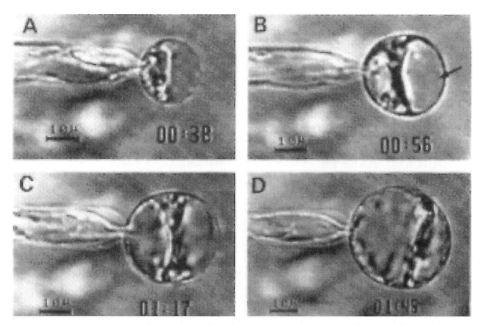

**Fig. 42:** *Laser microsurgery of a root hair of Medigaco sativa. After cutting the tip of the root hair, the protoplast is expelled by internal pressure.*

For all cell types protocols were developed which allowed the preparation of free membranes even at moderate laser powers. In spite of the fact that the membranes appeared to be very smooth, however, it was surprisingly difficult to get a good electric seal between patch-pipette and membrane, which is mandatory to measure correctly the tiny electric currents which are flowing through a single membrane channel molecule. Since similar diffculties were encountered after micromechanical membrane preparation, however, this may not be a specific problem of the laser technique but due to a general feature of these cell membranes. Nevertheless, two variants of patch clamping, the suction method and the electric break-through method, were partially successful and the opening and closing of membrane channels could be observed.

According to this study, one reason for the difficulties in obtaining a good electrical seal may be the fact that, when the cell wall is removed by laser pulses the plasmolyzed cell expands (as was seen quite dramatically for *Medigaco sativa*) and water flows out. Thereby debris of the cell wall or from elsewhere may be rinsed onto the cell membrane and stick there. For *Eremosphera* also another effect may prevent good seals: there some strand-like structures (Hechtian strands), which in the intact plant tissue serve as wall to membrane linkers, may be disrupted by the laser treatment and again the debris may settle down on the membrane. It remains to be seen whether measures against these two effects will improve the establishment of Mega-seals required for optimal patch clamping studies.

## Summary and outlook

A number of preparation techniques involving micro- or nanosurgery can be performed with the laser microbeam and supported by optical tweezers. Generally, this contact-free type of micromanipulation is gentler and often more versatile than mechanical microtools.

## Selected literature

A.H. de Boer, B. van Duijn, P. Giesberg, L. Wegner, G. Obermeyer, W. Köhler and K.W. Linz (1994) Laser microsurgery: A versatile tool in plant (electro) physiology. Protoplasma 178, 1-10.

K.O. Greulich, U. Bauder, S. Monajembashi, N. Ponelies, S. Seeger and J. Wolfrum (1989) UV Laser Mikrostrahl und optische Pinzette (UV laser microbeam and optical tweezers). Labor 2000, 36–42.

A. Kurkdjian, G. Leitz, P. Manigault, A. Harim and K.O. Greulich (1993) Non-enzymatic access to the plasma membrane of Medicago root hairs by laser microsurgery. J. Cell Science 105, 263–268.

G. Leitz, K.O. Greulich and E. Schnepf (1994) Laser microsurgery and optical trapping in the marine dinophyte *Pyrocystis noctiluca*. Botan. Acta 107, 90-94.

G. Leitz, E. Schnepf, K.O. Greulich (1995) Micromanipulation of statoliths in gravity sensing *Chara rhizoids* by optical tweezers. Planta, 197.2, 278- 288.

# 6.2 Microperforation of cell walls and cell membranes

### 6.2.1 Laser-microinjection: What do biologists want to know

There are many reasons why a biologist would wish to inject foreign material into cells or subcellular structures. Many substances can just be added to the culture medium and the cell will take them up spontaneously after a certain period. Often, however, an experiment may require the uptake of foreign material at a definite time, and also with a definite dose. In that case direct microinjection is the method of choice. One example would be the injection of fluorescently labeled molecules at a given time in order to study the temporal course of their distribution over the cell or their degradation with time. A second example is the introduction of caged compounds into cells for signal transduction research. In this case, ions essential for the initiation of signaling inside a cell are bound (caged) to other molecules such as DM nitrophen. In such a caged state the ions are inactive. After they have been injected into the cell the ions are liberated by a short light pulse and start, for example, a calcium wave for intracellular signaling or a cascade of intracellular motions. The injected material may also be a DNA molecule and this can be used to transfer genes into a target cell.

Probably the most efficient direct microinjection technique uses a fine glass capillary which pricks a hole into the cell membrane and allows one to directly inject the material. There are, however, some contraindications for using this micromechanical technique (Box 79). In some of these cases laser microinjection is the tool of choice.

**Box 79: Some contraindications for micromechanical injection of materials into cells**

- Holes are too large, viability is decreased
- Hard cell walls (plant cells), capillary breaks
- Molecule to be injected adheres to the capillary
- Cells are in suspension
- Internal pressure in the cell
- Steric hindrance by other cells
- Large number of cells per time has to be injected
- Microinjection into subcellular structures required

Laser microperforation is straightforward. The laser microbeam is directed toward the cell wall or cell membrane and with a short single pulse of high intensity it is perforated. The hole size depends on the laser intensity and may range from being virtually invisible to causing the destruction of the complete cell. Small holes in the membrane will reseal spontaneously after some time. This resealing time depends on temperature and is typically a few tenths of a second at 37 degrees Celsius, a few seconds at room temperature, and a few days at a temperature close to the freezing point of water. Thus one has two parameters which allow the microinjection of a vast variation of molecule types and a vast variation of molecule numbers. A third parameter is the osmotic pressure difference which can be modified by adding substances such as mannitol to the solvent. In order to determine optimal conditions it is necessary to perform some test experiments with any new cell type to be microinjected, but once the conditions have been determined, large numbers of cells (up to one per second) can be treated.

Since the laser microbeam works in a contact free way, it is no problem to perforate cells in suspension. This is a distinct advantage as compared to micoinjection with a glass capillary, which would tend to push suspension cells away instead of perforating them and thus in most cases requires adherently growing cells.

As an example of the possible accuracy of laser microperforation, Fig. 43 shows a human red blood cell with a pattern found on the surface of its membrane.

For good practical work the focus of the microbeam is adjusted exactly into the object plane. It is also helpful, though not mandatory, that the laser be focused close to the diffraction limit. For pricking holes into the cell surface it is only necessary to bring the cell surface in the focal plane, i.e. to obtain a sharp image of it. With a single pulse the hole is punched into the cell surface and material can slip into the cytoplasma. The hole size is highly dependent on the laser power.

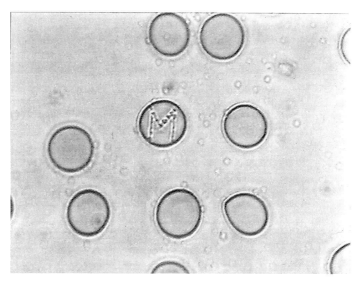

**Fig. 43:** *Pattern written on the surface of a human red blood cell.*

## 6.2.2 Laser-assisted gene transfer into animal cells

The first experiments on laser-facilitated gene transfer were performed with animal and human cells (Tsukakoshi et al., 1984; Kurata et al., 1986, Tao et al., 1987).

Plasmid DNA containing the gene for the enzyme "gpt" (pSV 2 gpt, ecogpt) was injected by a laser microbeam (third harmonic of an NdYAG laser) into normal rat kidney cells (NRK). Gpt converts xanthine into xantine-monophosphate and is thought to confer resistance against the action of substances inhibiting metabolism. After irradiation, the cultures were selected for 100 hours on medium containing antimetabolites. Survivors were found only when, before selection, the cells had received laser pulses in the presence of plasmid DNA. When, under continuous observation in the microscope, one half of the cells in the field of view was treated with the laser while the other half remained untreated, growth was observed only in the treated half. Transfection efficiencies up to 0.6% have been reported for this system (Tsukakoshi et al., 1984; Kurata et al., 1986).

In a similar experiment resistance to the aminoglycoside antibiotic G 418 was transferred to a human fibrosarcoma cell line by injection of the "neo" gene. The fibrosarcoma cell is deficient in the gene for hypoxanthine phospho-ribosyltransferase (HPRT) and should not grow in a medium containing G 418. When 1000 of

### Box 80: Gene transfer: Indirect bulk techniques

There are some techniques available to make cell membranes permeable for DNA. For example, some are based on the fact that cells take up DNA in the presence of calcium phosphate. An other approach is electroporation. Here, cells are placed into a pulsed electric field. The field pulses cause membrane permeabilization. DNA can slip into the cytoplasma through the holes in the membranes. In bacterial cells, as well as in other prokaryotes lacking a nucleus, the DNA can then be immediately inserted into the genome by the cell's own enzyme machinery.

In cells with nucleus the experience is that DNA can also reach the genome, albeit with lower efficiency.

Therefore, more direct techniques are desirable. Direct capillary injection is the most precise method but has its limitations (see above). It works well, for example, with adherently growing fibroblasts or cells such as the PtK2 cell used in other experiments described in this book, since they are flat and there is little cytoplasma between outer cell membrane and nuclear membrane. Direct microinjection is difficult or impossible with more spherical cells and particularly with cells in suspension, where the glass capillary tends to push the cell away rather than perforate it. In such cases one needs a second microtool to hold the cell to be injected. While this is possible, the process requires considerable experimental skill and only a small number of cells can be microinjected in a given time.

### Box 81: Southern blots

In a Southern blot the whole DNA of the cell is separated electrophoretically in a gel according to size. Then the gel is immersed in a suspension containing a labeled DNA probe for the gene under investigation (in this case it was the neo gene). When the latter is incorporated in the genome of the cell to be tested it will hybridize to the gel and thus label the neo gene. In cells not carrying this gene, no labeling will be observed.

### Box 82: Gene transfer into plant cells by *Agrobacterium tumefaciens*

A quite successful standard technique is to use the bacterium *Agrobacterium tumefaciens* as a carrier. However, it does not work equally well for all plant types. A number of other techniques exist, but they either do not allow targeted transfer into a selected cell or they have a low efficiency.

these cells were perforated by the laser microbeam in the presence of 12 µg/µl of a plasmid carrying the neo gene, three resistant colonies were detected (i.e. the transformation efficiency was 0.3%). In control experiments no colonies were found. Also, Southern blot analysis and microcell hybridization indicated that the gene indeed was incorporated.

The transformation efficiencies in both types of experiments, 0.3 to 0.6%, appear to be poor but clearly exceed transformation efficiencies of chemical methods. In addition, the laser technique has the advantage of microscopic control. In plant cell experiments it will turn out that even higher transformation efficiencies can be obtained.

### 6.2.3 Direct microinjection of genes into plant cells: The laser microbeam is often without alternative

While for animal cells direct transfer of genetic material by a glass capillary is a technique that competes with laser microinjection, with plant cells it is often no alternative. (Weber et al 1988 a and b, 1989). For example, when one tries to microinject material into cells of rapeseed, the capillaries are either too thick and damage the cell or they are sufficiently fine but too fragile and thus cannot penetrate the rigid plant cell wall. Although walls may be removed enzymatically, only in a few cases can those protoplasts be regenerated to plants.

Laser holes in membranes of cells of rapeseed (Weber et al., 1989 and 1990a) and, in an additional experiment, of tobacco (Weber et al 1990 b) were recorded on video. A fluorescent dye was taken up through laser holes into plasmolyzed cells for less than 5 seconds. Within ca. 5 seconds after irradiation they were closed. However, lowered membrane fluidity at temperatures below 11°C prevented the self-healing of laser holes. After irradiation, 80% of single cells were viable. One day later 40% of cells were alive and continued to grow. 24 hours after laser treatment the gene was expressed.

In developing embryos of rapeseed the expression of GUS (see Box 83) and its time course was followed. When GUS DNA was injected into some selected cells of the embryo, only the laser treated cells assumed a blue color indicating the successful expression of GUS.

More difficult, but with a wider field of applications, is the injection of foreign genes into individual cells in suspension. Single rapeseed cells were plasmolyzed

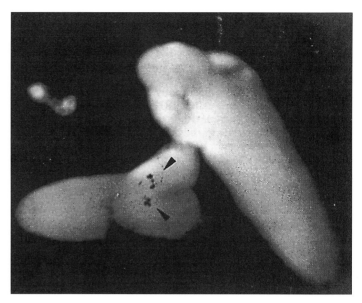

**Fig. 44:** *Expression of GUS in those cells of a rapeseed embryo, which were treated with the laser microbeam. On the right: A totally untreated embryo.*

to 80% of their volume in the presence of DNA conveying resistance to the antibiotic hygromycin (pRT 102 hph). After laser perforation of their cell wall, approximately $1 \times 10^6$ molecules were incorporated into each cell at a DNA concentration of 1 µg/µl. In one hour 1000 cells could be irradiated. Approximately 20% of the cells became resistant to the hygromycin and retained their resistance over many cell generations in the absence of selection.

**Box 83 The GUS reporter gene**

A number of gene constructs have become commercially available to monitor whether a gene is expressed after DNA transfer into a cell. One such reporter gene is bacterial glucuronidase (GUS) with the 35 S promoter of cauliflower mosaic virus. This promotor guarantees that the gene becomes active in its new host cell, irrespective of the position of integration into the plant genome.

Similar experiments with tobacco cells showed that from a total of 472 irradiated cells 2 fertile plants were regenerated which had the entire hph/gene incorporated into their genome. i.e. the transformation efficiency for *stable* incorporation is 0.5% (Fig. 44).

Stable incorporation of hph gene was also observed in tobacco. DNA of leaves from the plant was isolated and separated according to size by electrophoresis. A labeled hph DNA probe successfully hybridizes against the DNA of the tobacco leaf, indicating that the gene is still in the plant of the second daughter generation. In control plants, no hybridization is detected.

### 6.2.4 Injection of DNA into isolated chloroplasts and into chloroplasts within a plant cell

Chloroplasts (5 to 10 μm in diameter) are the organelles where photosynthesis occurs. They are particularly attractive targets for introducing DNA with the help of a laser microbeam. Chloroplasts of higher plants have their own DNA in the form of circular molecules. Typically, several DNA copies are present in one chloroplast. Similarly as the genomic DNA in the nucleus, chloroplast DNA codes for proteins. Interestingly, the enzyme machinery used for protein synthesis resembles that of prokaryotic bacteria.

In a first experiment, the membrane of isolated chloroplasts was opened with single laser shots. Compared to irradiating cell walls, the laser pulse energy had to be attenuated in order to prevent bursting of the chloroplasts. Furthermore, the integrity of the entire chloroplast was critically dependent on exact focusing of the laser. For scoring a hit of the membrane a visible effect was recorded (Weber et al., 1990b).

For injection of foreign genes into the chloroplast it was essential that a hole in its membrane sealed approximately 1 second after laser treatment. The small diameter of the focus (less than 1 μm) and its small depth of field made it possible to aim a laser at the membrane of chloroplasts *inside* of cells. DNA was transferred into chloroplasts by microinjection into the cytoplasm of the protoplasts, i.e. rape-

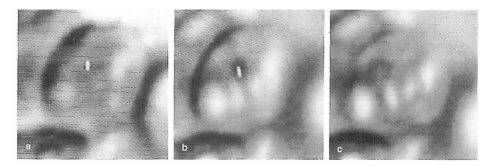

**Fig. 45:** *Generation of laser holes on the surface of isolated chloroplasts inside an unopened cell.*

221

seed cells whose cell wall was digested enzymatically. Then the laser was aimed at individual chloroplasts inside of the cytoplasm. In this way fluorescently-labeled DNA was introduced into chloroplasts.

One marker gene for chloroplasts is the gene psbA. In the presence of triacines which are usually lethal, cells containing this gene are capable of performing photosynthesis. 1000 protoplasts were loaded with plasmid DNA carrying psbA. Within 30 min all visible chloroplasts received one laser pulse. Two weeks later selection on atrazine was started and resistant, green colonies grew from laser-treated cells indicating transient expression of the resistance marker psbA. The colonies were picked and then followed through two more rounds of selection. Finally 16 resistant colonies remained from the 1000 cells initially irradiated. However, in this case, no resistant plants could be regenerated.

## Summary and outlook

Cell membranes and cell walls can be easily perforated with the laser microbeam. This can be used for laser-assisted gene transfer into animal and particularly into plant cells. Microperforation of subcellular structures residing in their natural environment, i.e. inside a living cell, is also possible with the laser microbeam. Here, the laser technique has no equal.

## Selected literature

S.I. Kurata, M. Tsukakoshi, T. Kasuya and Y. Ikawa (1986) Laser method for efficient introduction of foreign DNA into cultured tissue cells. Exp. Cell Res. 162, 372378.

K. Schütze, H.-D. Reiss, H. Becker, S. Monajembashi and K.O. Greulich (1989) Laser microsurgery on pollen tubes Ber. Bunsenges. Phys. Chem. 93, 249.

M. Tsukakoshi, S. Kurata, Y. Nomiya Y. Ikawa and T. Kasuya (1984) A new method of DNA transfection by laser microbeam cell surgery. Appl. Phys. B. 35, 135–140.

W. Tao, J. Wilkinson, E.J. Stanbridge and M.W. Berns (1987) Directed gene transfer into human cultured cells facilitated by laser micropuncture of the cell membranes Proc. Natl. Acad. Sci. 84, 4180–4184.

G. Weber, S. Monajembashi, K. O. Greulich and J. Wolfrum (1988) Injection of DNA into plant cells using a UV laser microbeam. Naturwissenschaften 75, 36.

G. Weber, S. Monajembashi, K.O. Greulich and J. Wolfrum (1988) Genetic manipulation of plant cells and organelles with a microfocused laser beam. Plant Cell, Tissue and Organ Culture 12, 219.

G. Weber, S. Monajembashi, J. Wolfrum and K.O. Greulich (1989a) Uptake of DNA in chloroplasts of Brassica napus (L) facilitated by a UV laser microbeam. Eur. J. Cell Biol. 49, 73.

G. Weber, S. Monajembashi, J. Wolfrum and K.O. Greulich (1989b) A laser microbeam as a tool to introduce genes into cells and organelles of higher plants. Ber. Bunsenges. Phys. Chem. 93, 252.

G. Weber, S. Monajembashi, J. Wolfrum and K.O. Greulich (1990a) Genetic changes induced in higher plant cells by a laser microbeam. Physiologia Plantarum 79, 190-193.

G. Weber, S. Monajembashi, K.O. Greulich and J. Wolfrum (1990b) Genetic changes induced in higher plants by a UV laser microbeam. Israel J. Botany 40, 115–122.

## 6.3 From laser-induced cell fusion to antibodies and immunology

In the section on the development of the roundworm *Caenorhabditis elegans* an experiment was reported whereby cells in an embryo were fused and their fate was subsequently studied (Schierenberg, 1984). This technique was later applied successfully by Clement Sengewald et al. (1993) in mammalian embryos. Two cell stage embryos of mice and cattle oocyte-cytoplast complexes were fused and their fate was studied. The fusion of two cells required up to one hour. So far only the feasibility of this process has been studied, no further applications are known. In the following sections a different type of cell fusion will be discussed: individual cells in suspension are fused with the help of a few short laser pulses.

## 6.3.1 How to avoid sex: Cell fusion in suspension

Genetic modification of a cell or an organism can be performed by introducing a defined gene into a target cell by, for example, laser microinjection (Section 6.2). Such a gene transfer modifies the target in one or a few specific traits, for example it can make a plant resistant to a specific disease. A more general way is the fusion of different cell types with each other, thus combining their two genomes in a similar way as it happens during sexual reproduction.

Spontaneous fusion of somatic (non-germline) cells is observed in muscle cells forming myofibrils. Other spontaneous cell fusions in an organism are unwanted since they may cause cancer. On the other hand, *in vitro* fusion of cells has now become an important tool in basic research and in biotechnology, since fusion allows one to generate variability at a speed which is often considerably larger than sexual reproduction in, for example, classical breeding. Unlike gene transfer, fusion allows modification of cellular properties in cases where a relevant gene is not known, i.e. when one works on a phenomenological basis.

Several techniques for the induction of cell fusion *in vitro* are available:

1   chemically induced cell fusion, particularly by polyethyleneglycol,
2   virus-induced cell fusion, particularly by *Sendai* virus,
3   fusion by electric microsecond field pulses, and
4   fusion by mechanically pricking adjacent cells.

Chemically- and virus-induced fusion are essentially mass fusion techniques. Large amounts of two cell types are mixed in suspension, the fusing agent is added and spontaneous fusion under these physicochemical condition are exploited. There will be fusions between cells of equal type (which in most cases are unwanted) and fusions between cells of different types. Usually a selection system guarantees that only the fusion products of different cell types will survive. Often, resistance against antibiotics is used as a marker for selection. When, for example, a long-living cell which is sensitive to an antibiotic is mixed with a resistant short-living cell, then fusion products of the short-living cell will die out naturally, those of the long living cell will die due to their sensitivity to the antibiotic. Fusion products of both cell types, however, may be long-living *and* resistant, i.e. they will have a massive growth advantage and will finally survive

Electrofusion is either a mass fusion technique (as it is used in most cases) or a technique for individual cells. In the latter case, however, complicated geometries of the electric field are required. Finally, mechanical fusion uses microtools to press or to prick cells and thereby induce their fusion. Both techniques for the fusion of individual cells are tedious. Here the laser may be the tool of choice.

When the laser microbeam is slightly defocused it will not longer burn holes into the membranes of mammalian cells or cut subcellular structures as it was described in Sections 5.4 and 6.2. When two cells are in contact with each other, they may be fused by a short series of laser pulses. Thus it is possible to fuse a pair of cells under total microscopic control. One can even select a specific region of a cell membrane where fusion should be induced.

The contact between cells involved in the fusion process may be established either by adhesive forces, due to high cell density on a microscope slide or by specific coupling via a bridging molecule system such as avidin/biotin.

### 6.3.2 Fusion of plant protoplasts

The perspective for fusing plant cells is that of accelerating plant breeding. Classical plant breeding is dependent on generation times which may last a year or more. Also, while it is possible to cross quite different plants with each other, in some cases a barrier of unknown origin prevents the combination of two specific traits.

Also, it is not possible to fuse plant *cells* with each other. Protoplasts first have to be generated by digestion of the hard cell wall with an enzyme cocktail. In this sense plant cell fusion is different from laser-induced gene transfer, since the latter also works with whole cells. Nevertheless, while protoplasts are more fragile than cells, viable fusion products can be obtained with reasonable yield.

Fig. 46 shows how protoplasts of the oilseed *Brassica napus* L. are fused. They were brought onto the microscope slide at high density. Since the protoplasts have a slight tendency to aggregate anyway, many pairs or even groups of three protoplasts can be found. The pair to be fused is brought into the focus of the laser microbeam. The laser is focused at the approximate location of contact area of the membranes of the cells. Then a series of laser pulses is released. After perturbing the protoplast membranes both protoplasts typically fuse their membranes forming a single cell after 10 to 20 s. During the release of the laser pulses it is often necessary to change the focal plane slightly in order to perturbate the membrane properly.

After fusion of the first two protoplasts was completed, a third protoplast was fused with the product of the first experiment. In principle this process can be repeated further, thus obtaining large multi-nucleated protoplasts.

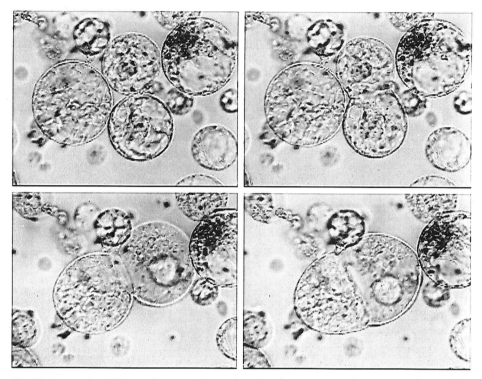

**Fig. 46:** *Laser induced fusion of rapeseed protoplasts. In a first step, two adjacent protoplasts in the center of the figure are fused. In a second step, the large protoplast to the left is fused to the hybrid product of the first step. In total a hybrid of three cells is generated.*

Initiation of membrane fusion as well as its progress is typically recorded on video tape. The analysis of individual video frames reveals details of the fusion mechanism. The following results were obtained after inspection of a series of different fusion events.

Protoplasts in close proximity before laser treatment show normal membrane features (Fig. 46a). When the membrane of only one cell was perturbated with the laser, it fused with the membrane of the adjacent cell. However, fusion of the cytoplasm did not occur. Instead, a bulge of the membrane of the presumably intact cell protruded into the cytoplasm of the opened cell (Fig. 46b). Eventually the plasmalemma of the intact cell ruptured to complete the fusion process (Fig. 46c). However, it is also possible to complete fusion by puncturing the remaining plasma membrane with additional laser pulses.

The yield of surviving hybrids can be checked by observing cytoplasmic streaming. This continued in more than 50% of the fusion products for at least one hour after membrane fusion.

### 6.3.3 Why single-cell fusion? Some speculation

The reason why fusion under total microscopic control is desirable becomes particularly evident in hybridoma research. Hybridoma are fusion products of B cells, those immune cells which have the potential to produce antibodies, with myeloma cells, a sort of blood cancer cells. In order to produce a specific monoclonal antibody against a certain antigen, typically a mouse is injected with this antigen and develops an immune response. B cells specific for the antigen are enriched and may make up to 5% of all B cells in the immune system of this particularly immunized mouse. Then the mouse is sacrificed. Its the spleen, the organ where B cells are highly enriched, is used to prepare the B cells. They are fused in a mass procedure, PEG- or electro-fusion (see Section 6.3.1) with the myeloma cells. Only then, following a complicated screening process often requiring months, is the hybridoma with the potential to produce antibodies of one or a few single specificities, selected from the mixture of many specificities.

Apart from the disadvantage of the lengthy preparation procedure, the antibodies are difficult to use in human therapy since, being derived from a mouse, they are recognized by the human immune system as alien and an immune response is mounted against the therapeutic antigen. This is one reason why, so far, antibody-based therapies have not become clinical routine.

What follows is speculation, not experimental results. It is suggested how some of the problems with antibody therapies might be overcome, based on the possibility of fusing a given pair of cells under total microscopic control, the subject has already been broached in this chapter in connection with laser techniques.

At any given time, the human immune system contains 150000 million B cells with the potential to produce 10 million different antibodies (each cell can produce only one type of antibody). Only 15000 cells are available for each specificity.

This is terribly little, particularly when a sample of, say, 100 ml of blood is to be used as the source to isolate B cells for hybrydoma production. In such cases one can expect to find only a few hundred B cells with a given specifity. In order to have a chance at all to get a few hybridoma, a fusion technique is required which has a high yield. Note, however, that this speculative strategy does not require immunization. We are just selecting from a large and highly variant pool. Since peripheral blood may be used, it is conceivable to produce an antibody for a human being using that individual's own immune cells as starting material – this certainly has the potential to alleviate many of the problems mentioned above for therapy.

So far the speculation. Let us come now back to reality. What is the state of the art on the way to hybridoma production under total microscopic control?

### 6.3.4 Laser-induced fusion of B cells with myeloma cells

As mentioned above the aim of hybrodoma technology is to produce a long-living antibody-producing cell by fusion of a short-living B lymphocyte with a long-living myeloma cell. Fig. 47 (from Wiegand et al., 1987) shows schematically how high specificity can be achieved.

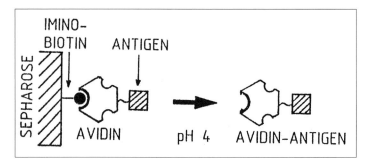

**Fig. 47:** *Fusion of two cells coupled by an antigen avidin biotin bridge. Schematic representation of the bridge.*

The two cells to be fused have been coupled by a specific process. An antigen (keyhole limpet protein, KLH) has been coupled to streptavidin. This construct can bind specifically to B cells specific for KLH. As a consequence, KLH-specific B cells, but no other B cells carry streptavidin at their surface. The trick is now to label myeloma cells with biotin, which is possible just by mixing. Due to the high affinity between biotin and streptavidin, the biotin labeled myeloma cells now bind preferentially to the avidin-labeled, KLH specific B cells. In other words, the cells with the wanted specificity are now implicitly marked and they are in the correct spatial situation for laser induced fusion.

The fusion is induced by a series of laser pulses similar to that described above for the plant protoplasts. In contrast to the latter, the fusion, i.e. the rounding of the fusion product, is completed after 10 minutes.

The specificity can be shown directly by using a fluorescently labeled antigen: By fluorescence labeling this single cell can be made visible among millions of B lymphocytes with other specificities, brought into contact with a myeloma cell and fused with laser pulses.

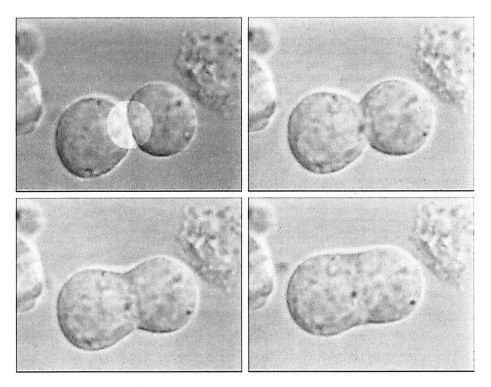

**Fig. 48:** *Fusion of two myeloma cells. The whole process takes approx. 10 min.*

### Box 84: Antibodies. Variability, reaction and production

#### Variability

Antibodies are produced by activated B lymphocytes (plasma cells). Each B lymphocyte can produce only one type of antibody, though many copies of it. At any time, there are some 100 million different antibodies in the human repertoire, and at any given time the human body has a repertoire of approx. 10 million different antibodies available to defeat disease. Since man has only 75–80000 genes it is clear that the variability has to be generated by some combinatorics. The immune system's trick is a combination of a few components of antibodies (light and heavy variable chain, light and heavy constant chain, joining region), each of which is coded by only a limited number of different genes (alleles). Additional variability is guaranteed by somatic mutation. It is likely that an individual can generate new antibody types even at an advanced age, and certainly the immune response via antibodies can be "trained".

### Reaction

Antibodies recognize bacteria, parasites or hazardous molecules (antigens) and bind to them with their variable regions. Their constant parts are then recognized by other cells of the immune system which incorporate and digest the antigen and the antibody bound to it, thereby eliminating the antigen from the body. But they do not only eat them away. They also use parts of the incorporated antibody to present them to T helper cells which then orchestrate the amplification of those B cells which can produce exactly this antibody. The result is that a few days after infection a large number of antibody producing B cells and antibodies are available to eliminate the antigen. This process of generating antibodies and their relevant B lymphocytes can be induced in a controlled way by injecting the antigen. When the antigen is a molecule or a virus, one can inject a few micrograms of slightly modified forms which are not as virulent but provoke a similar immune response. This is vaccination. Since the antibody repertoire is so large, many antibodies will recognize the antigen, some in a more efficient way, some only marginally. The production of such a mixture of antibodies is called a polyclonal response.

### Production

When one specific (monoclonal) antibody type is required, often mice are immunized with antigen. Their spleen, an organ containing B cells in high concentration, is isolated and B cells are cultivated individually, i.e. they are cloned. Unfortunately B cells die after a few cell divisions. They have to be immortalized by fusion with long living blood cancer cells (myeloma). The result can be a long living, antibody producing cell, a hybridoma. The present strategy is first to create a large number of hybridoma in a mass fusion and then to select in a lengthy screening process for the one hybridoma producing the best monoclonal antibody against the antigen under investigation. An alternative strategy would be first to select the B cell with the potential to produce the wanted antibody, immortalize it by fusion and then to grow it in culture.

## 6.3.5 Increasing the laser fusion yield by chemicals

At present, laser-induced fusion of such a cell pair can be induced with a yield of approximately 20%. This can be increased to 40% when 1% polyethyleneglycol (PEG) is added to the solution. Such a PEG concentration is far below typical values in classical PEG fusion experiments and for that reason much less toxic. Spontaneous cell fusion solely by 1% PEG does not occur. Until now only the biophysical process of formation of hybrid cells has been studied but so far it has been difficult to recover hybrid cell clones. It still has to be shown that those clones are the result of the fusion process and not just spontaneous clones resulting from a mutation. Laser-induced cell fusion is not restricted to comparatively large mammalian or plant cells. Originally, it was detected in protoplasts of baker's yeast. An additional advantage of laser-induced cell fusion is that cells or protoplasts of different size can be fused. This is sometimes difficult with other physical techniques such as electrofusion. The mechanism of laser-induced fusion has not yet been elucidated in detail. However, there appear to be differences from electrofusion. An electric field perforates the cell membranes in the area of contact between two adjacent cells thereby inducing the fusion process. In laser fusion occasionally a membrane remains within the fusion product

This indicates that there is no large scale perforation of membrane material, but that the laser perturbs the involved membranes in a more subtle way and surface tension causes the reorganization of the membranes. The separating membrane can be disrupted by a laser pulse targeted onto this structure in the depth of the newly formed hybrid cell. For some basic studies in cell biology it may be desirable to keep the separating membrane intact. This would be a further application of laser-induced cell fusion since such a task is difficult to perform using other techniques.

A further observation hinting at the mechanism is the linear relationship between membrane potential and fusion yield when two myeloma cells are fused in the laser microbeam

Though this observation is not yet quantitatively understood, it is obvious that electromechanical properties of the cell membrane are relevant in the process of laser-induced cell fusion.

### 6.3.6 Increasing the yield by combining laser microbeam and optical tweezers

A very elegant method to increase the yield of laser-induced suspension fusion is to combine laser microbeam and optical tweezers. Then one can avoid any natural or chemically-induced contact. Any pair of cells visible under the microscope can be brought into contact, as in the manner shown for the attack of NK cells on blood cancer cells in Section 5.1. Once they are in contact, fusion can be induced as described in Section 6.3.5. In an experiment reported by Wiegand Steubing et al. (1991) a nitrogen-pumped dye laser (wavelength 366 nm) was used to induce the fusion process. Box 85 summarizes the results.

**Box 85: Efficiency of laser-induced cell fusion in culture medium (tyr/trp – RPMI)**

| | Cells trapped and irradiated | Cell pairs fused | Efficiency |
|---|---|---|---|
| 0% PEG | 75 | 1 | 1.3% |
| 0.1% PEG, 25 °C | 112 | 9 | 8.6% |
| 0.1% PEG, 37 °C | 54 | 6 | 11.0% |

For the cell type used in this fusion experiment (with the myeloma cell line NS1) the addition of PEG is obviously essential, since without PEG only one fusion has been observed. The PEG concentration required is still very small as compared to the conventional PEG technique and the fusion can still be induced under laser control. This preserves the high degree of microcopic control which had been observed in the other laser cell fusion experiments described above.

### 6.3.7 Optical tweezers-based immunosensors and detectors of virus-cell adhesion

Laser microbeams and optical tweezers are used not only in antibody *production* but also in antibody *detection*. For example, when antibodies and antigens are bound on the surface of microspheres the force between the spheres can be measured as has already been described (see particularly Sections 5.1 and 5.2). With good assumptions on the density of antigen respectively antibody densities on the spheres the force between single molecules can be estimated. Since there is a relationship between force and binding constant, such an experiment gives also information about the antigen-antibody binding constant. With these mechanisms in mind, an optical tweezers-based immunosensor has been constructed (Helmerson et al., 1997). Any other system of molecules and macromolecular complexes can be similarly studied quite easily. An example of considerable practical importance is the study of virus-cell adhesion and, particularly, the effects of inhibitors thereof, which might be used as protectors against virus infection. In this case a microsphere is coated with virus particles and its adhesion to cells is studied by a double optical tweezers system which is called OPTCOL since it allows one to study optically-controlled collisions of biological objects (Mammen et al., 1996).

### 6.3.8 Optical tweezers reveal details of the attack on the immune system on cancer

The following experiment (Seeger et al., 1991) describes how, with the help of optical tweezers, the attack of a cell from the human immune system on a cancer cell can be observed from the very first seconds after contact has been established. Immune cells such as cytotoxic T lymphocytes (CTL) and natural killer (NK) cells circulate through the body and check if other cells show for example signs of cancer. Usually, cells present peptides bound to a molecule class called MHC 1. If such a peptide is unfamiliar to the CTL it attacks the presenting cell. If for some reason the presenting cell has no MHC 1 molecule at all, it cannot present the peptide which might indicate that something is wrong. In that case, the NK cell takes over the task of immune surveillance and thus helps to avoid a catastrophic outcome for the whole organism. In order to understand the process of recognition and attack, *in vitro* experiments would be helpful, where contact is established artificially and the process can be observed. Particularly interesting is the contact between cytolytic effector cells such as cytotoxic T lymphocytes (CTLs) or natural killer cells (NKs) with target cells. The CTL-target contact is highly specific and governed by complex supramolecular associations between T cell receptor and CD 8 surface molecules on the effector cell and major histocompatibility class I surface molecules complexed with peptides on the target cell. With NK cells similar mechanisms have been suggested. In order to test such working hypotheses, it is helpful to have other techniques for establishing contact between NK cell and its target cell.

The standard approach is to mix the two types of cells, centrifuge them at low speed and observe what happens after the cells have been resuspended and prepared for microscopy or for other experiments. This approach is blind for the first minutes after contact between the two reaction partners and therefore cannot study the most important phase of the attack. Alternatively, contact can be established by use of micromechanical tools, but this may damage the NK cells and thus blur the outcome of the experiment. Here the optical trap can establish contact in an easy and gentle way. With the optical tweezers, the NK cell can be moved towards its target

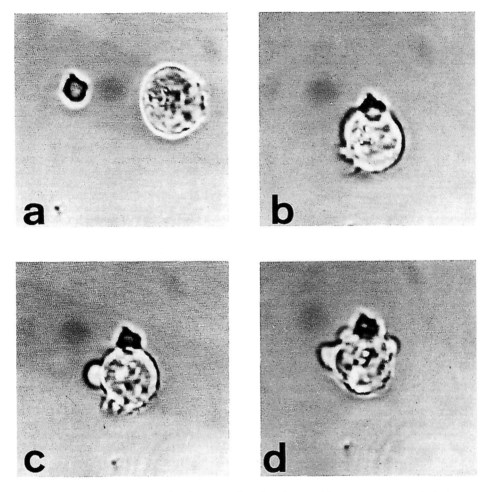

**Fig. 49:** *Attack of a NK cell on a blood cancer cell, induced by establishing contact with the help of optical tweezers*

cell and even the natural contact between both cells can be increased. This may help to trigger the activity of the target cell. During such experiments the yield of successful attacks of NK cells on erythroleukemia cells was higher than expected from literature values. An obvious explanation is that the NK attack on the target cells has already started when the affinity of recognizing molecules per se is not sufficiently high to trigger activation. In these cases supporting the contact by the optical tweezers may support activation even in those cases, where specific contact is not yet fully established. Fig. 49 shows that the NK cell (small dark cell) in fact attacks the target cell, which changes its morphology by membrane blebbing.

A detailed inspection of membrane blebbing shows that for the first 40 to 50 seconds after contact between NK and cancer cells no change in morphology is observed. This can be explained by biochemical activation processes which take some time before the cancer cell really is attacked. The further process, interestingly, is not continuous but oscillating. At present this oscillation is unexplained. A speculative interpretation would be that the attacked cell reacts by repairing damage and that the attacking cell increases its attempts to kill the cancer cell. If this interpretation turns out to be realistic, it would have significant consequences for the understanding of immune surveillance of cancers and might give interesting hints for developing cancer therapies.

## Summary and outlook

Laser-induced cell fusion is a convenient way to combine the genomes of a selected pair of cells. This is difficult to accomplish with any other cell fusion method. With the laser technique it is even possible to generate hybrids of a preselected number of cells, for example, a cell triplet. The immune attack of natural killer cells on a blood cancer cell can be induced by optical tweezers. In turn, the force between antigen and antibody can be measured and substances can be studied which modify virus-cell adhesion.

## Selected literature

A. Clement-Sengewald, K. Schütze, A. Heinze, G.A.Palme, H. Pösl and G. Brem (1993) Laser assisted cell fusion and cytoplastic transfer in early mammalian embryos. SPIE Proceedings Vol. 1876, 187–193.

K. Helmerson, R. Kishore, W.D. Phillips and H.H. Weetall (1997) Optical tweezers-based immunosensor detects femtomolar concentration of antigens. Clin. Chem. 43.2, 379–383.

M. Mammen, K. Helmerson, R. Kishore, S.K. Choi, W.D. Phillips and G.M. Whiteside (1996) Optically controlled collisions of biological objects to evaluate potent polyvalent inhibitors of virus-cell adhesion. Chem. Biol. 3.9, 757–763.

E. Schierenberg (1984) Altered cell division rates after laser induced cell fusion in nematode embryos. Dev. Biol. 101, 240–245.

S. Seeger, S. Monajembashi, K.-J. Hutter, G. Futtermann, J. Wolfrum and K.O. Greulich (1991) Application of laser optical tweezers in immunology and molecular genetics. Cytometry, 12, 497–504.

R. Wiegand, G. Weber, K. Zimmermann, S. Monajembashi, J. Wolfrum and K.O. Greulich (1987) Laser induced fusion of mammalian cells and plant protoplasts. J. Cell. Science 88, 145.

R. Wiegand-Steubing, S. Cheng, W.H. Wright, Y. Numajiri, M.W. Berns (1991) Laser induced cell fusion in combination with optical tweezers: The laser cell fusion trap. Cytometry, 505–510.

# 6.4 Towards medical diagnostics: From blood to cancer

The biomedical applications reported so far are still basic research. The techniques now discussed in this section are on their way to diagnostic applications. They deal with the elasticity of red blood cells for the diagnosis of blood circulation problems and with the isolation of selected cells from a cancer tissue, a technique which may soon contribute to an improved cancer diagnostics.

## 6.4.1 Optical tweezers as wall-free microvessels to study red blood cell elasticity

Red blood cells (erythrocytes), the transporters of oxygen in the organism, are special with respect to their cellular architecture. While typical animal cells have a cytoskeleton throughout their cytoplasm, red blood cells are stabilized by a skeleton of spectrin molecules immediately below the membrane. This membrane skeleton stiffens the membrane and determines its mechanical properties.

Red blood cells may be highly deformed when they are squeezed through narrow blood vessels and thus the mechanics of the spectrin-membrane system is a property of vital importance both for the cell and for the organism which they have to supply with oxygen. When red blood cells become too stiff, their transport through the finest capillaries of the human blood system is impeded and blood supply is blocked.

The study of red blood cell elasticity (a branch of Rheology), particularly the influence of physicochemical parameters such as salt concentration, by classical means is difficult since the cells somehow have to be held in a suitable position mechanically. This may deform the cells and thus affect their elasticity. Optical tweezers can alleviate a number of typical problems encountered with such elasticity studies since the red blood cells can be fixed by the comparatively gentle gradient forces. In a sense, the focus of the optical tweezers serves as a wall-free microvessel.

In the following, two types of experiments are reported. First, the elasticity of whole cells or whole membranes and their adhesion properties are investigated. Second, in order to bring to light more details, membrane skeletons are isolated from red blood cells and investigated separately without membrane material. Such a study allows one to directly ascertain the contribution of the skeleton to red blood cell stability.

## 6.4.2 Measuring the elasticity of red blood cells

Box 86 summarizes some non laser techniques used to study red blood cell elasticity.

### Box 86: Conventional techniques to study red blood cell flexibility

**Red cell filtration**

This technique simulates the situation in a blood vessel. The cells are forced through a filter membrane with suitable pore diameter. In a population of highly elastic cells a larger fraction will pass the filter than in a population of rigid cells.

**Micropipette**

In the micropipette technique a cell is partly aspired into one or two pipettes. After a sudden release of mechanical stress, shape revovery is measured.

**Rheoscope**

In the rheoscope cells are deformed by a linear shear flow of liquid. As in the micropipette method, shape recovery is measured.

Multibeam optical tweezers represent a gentle alternative to the technique described above (Bronkhorst et al., 1995). Red blood cells have a biconvex shape resembling a thick flexible disk of which the centers of the two faces are slightly pressed towards each other. In single beam tweezers the red blood cells would orient themselves always parallel to the direction of the laser beam. Triple beam tweezers allow one to orient the cell perpendicularly to the original direction. Using three partial laser beams, the membranes of the cells can be perturbed into shape resembling a parachute, or in a very crude approximation, into a V cross-section shape (Bronkhorst et al., 1995). Two beams pull two extreme parts of the cell. A third beam in the middle pushes the center away and thereby deforms the whole cell. After switching the lasers off, the cell relaxes into its original structure. The shape recovery is recorded on video tape and subsequently evaluated. For example, using video tape one can measure the time it takes for the relaxation process to be completed halfway. Approximately 50 cells per hour can be analyzed by way of this technique.

The relaxation is quantified as follows: The angle of the V-shaped cell which opens increasingly as the cell relaxes is plotted versus time and fitted by an exponential curve (or, more precisely, against a curve of the type (1-exp). From this the relaxation time or $T_{1/2}$ can be calculated similarly as it was discussed in Section 3.4.

From experiments using the micropipette and the rheoscope it is known that $T_{1/2}$ depends on the age of the red blood cells and this in turn is related to their density. Therefore, for the laser experiments the red blood cells were separated into two fractions with high and low densities (old and young cells) in a centrifuge, using the commercially available separation medium, Ficoll. Also, red blood cells in buffer have been compared with those in blood plasma (the liquid component of blood after removing all cellular components). The laser results are compared with literature values obtained by the two classical methods; however, in buffer only. Box 87 summarizes the results.

**Box 87: Elasticity of old and young human red blood cells, given as $T_{1/2}$ in milliseconds obtained by three different methods, including optical tweezers**

|  | Old cells | Young cells | Total |
|---|---|---|---|
| Optical tweezers, plasma | 360 | 180 | 290 |
| Optical tweezers, buffer | n.d. | n.d. | 100 |
| Micropipette, buffer | 100 | 80 | 90 |
| Rheoscope, buffer | 100 | 90 | 180 |

In spite of a few inconsistencies (with the rheoscope the value for all cells is higher than the average for old and young cells) the following picture emerges.

1  In blood plasma $T_{1/2}$ is much longer than in buffer. In order to come close to and in vivo situation, blood plasma has to be taken as solvent.

2  Where comparable, all methods give similar values for $T_{1/2}$ within a factor of two.

The overall result of these experiments is that triple beam optical tweezers prove suitable for measure the flexibility of red blood cells. It is obvious that this technique can be used immediately in clinical diagnostics of red blood cell properties.

### 6.4.3 Red cell adhesion: Laser tweezers test two models

As important as the elasticity of red blood cells is their tendency to form aggregates by adhesion. Bronkhorst et al (1997) used a double beam optical tweezers trap to induce two cell aggregates by pushing them towards each other. In a second step, these two cell aggregates were pulled apart and it was observed under the microscope that tethers formed. In addition it was difficult to pull the two cells apart in a direction perpendicular to the surface. Only a tangential motion with a speed of the order of micrometers per second allowed their separation. This is not consistent with a model for red blood cell adhesion which required steric exclusion of macromolecules and therefore confirms the "cross bridge" model which requires the formation of membrane tethers between the two adjacent cells.

### 6.4.4 Studies on the isolated membrane skeleton

Svoboda et al. (1992) devised a protocol for preparation and observation of isolated red blood cell membranes. In order to have a full microscopic control over the preparation process, as a first step, a silica bead (0.5 μm diameter) is coupled to a complete red blood cell. The cell with the bead is then introduced into a microscope flow chamber. By trapping the silica bead, the cell can be held in a flow streaming with an velocity of up to 100 mm/s. The solvent in the flow can be easily exchanged by exchanging the reservoirs supplying it. When the solvent contains a detergent (Triton X100) the membrane and intracellular structures are dissolved and rinsed away and one can observe under the microscope how the membrane skeleton remains coupled to the silica bead and trapped by the tweezers.

Immediately after extraction the buffer can be exchanged again and parameters such as the diameter or the surface area of the membrane skeleton can be recorded. A particularly simple empirical relationship was observed for dependence of the diameter d on salt concentration c (in mM)

$$d = \text{const} \cdot c^{-0.13} \approx \text{const} \cdot d^{-1/8}. \quad (36)$$

This equation is roughly valid for concentrations between 100 mM up to 2 M. The major result of this study is that free spectrin is surprisingly flexible. The length over which it appears stiff (the persistence length, see Box 60 in Section 5.1.5) at a salt concentration of 150 mM is only 10 nm, i.e., spectrin molecules shorter than this length appear as stiff rods while longer ones are more comparable to ropes which can, for example, form coils.

## 6.4.5 Tissue microdissection in cancer research: Background

The development of many cancers and probably other diseases can be regarded as an evolutionary process. Cells of a healthy tissue evolve by mutation, either due to spontaneous reading errors or through the influence of chemicals or radiation. Most of these mutations are neutral, i.e. they do not affect health. Others modify the cell to such a far degree that the immune system of the organism recognizes this and eliminates the erroneous cell. Only very occasionally are the changes small enough not to be recognized by the body's defense system but severe enough to remove growth constraints which usually guarantee that the cell remains within the social network of the tissue. When the cell starts to grow autonomously, this is the first step in the development of cancer.

A cancer tissue consists of cells with a wide variety of genetic outfits. As a consequence, a large number of cells may be still amenable to therapy but a small fraction may be refractive. This has been suggested to be the reason for an often observed time course of cancer therapies: the first stage of therapy appears to be successful, the tumor regresses. But at some stage the tumor recurs and cannot be treated further. When such a time course is compared with cases where no therapy was applied, it often turns out that the total time of survival of a patient is not very different. The untreatable cells have replaced those cells which were destroyed by the therapy. In order to find out which cells are the untreatable ones and what property makes them untreatable, individual cells are isolated from a cancer tissue. Their surface can be investigated by cancer-specific antibodies. For example, in Hodgkin's disease, only a small number of cells are really cancer cells. Only they can be stained with a cancer-specific antibody called CD 30. In this tumor it may be useful to isolate individual cells and to investigate if certain genes are expressed incorrectly or if they are mutated. Also, in virus-dependent cancers one may try to find out which cells are infected, i.e. in which cell specific genes of the virus are expressed. The molecular biological technique is the polymerase chain reaction.

A second motivation for attempting single cell analysis is the fact that in many hospitals a large amount of tissue sections of past cancer cases are available. They may be used for retrospective studies. Since this valuable archival material should not be destroyed as a whole, single-cell analysis gives the wanted information at minimal damage of the tissue.

### 6.4.6 Laser capture microdissection and laser pressure catapulting

The isolation of the single cell is often accomplished by mechanical microtools. However, with this technique cells may be damaged during the preparation procedure, and it is difficult to isolate single cells. Thus adjacent cells with a different genetic constitution may blur the results.

The potential of laser microsurgery for the isolation of single cells or groups of cells has been recognized early on and comparably sophisticated equipment has been developed (Meier-Ruge et al., 1976). A nitrogen laser focused to the diffraction limit was combined with a helium-neon laser of low power. The latter could be used to mark a region of cells in freeze-dried tissue slices by circumscribing the region to be microdissected at a later stage of the experiment. The data were stored electronically and subsequently the nitrogen laser performed the cutting work automatically.

An interesting technical variant is laser capture microdissection (LCM, Emmert-Buck et al., 1996). The tissue is covered with a thermoplastic film. By shining the laser onto the tissue region under study, the film is softened. The film can now be torn off and the tissue region is isolated. However, the diameter of the isolated region is larger than 50 μm and thus LCM at present is not a single-cell technique. In contrast, in a further variant, where the light pressure of the cutting laser is used to "blow" the desired cell out of the tissue (Schütze et al., 1997 a, b, Schütze and Lahr, 1998), single-cell isolation is possible (laser pressure catapulting).

So far, the different technical variants have not yet been compared with respect to efficiency. Only a few complete experiments in cancer research have been performed. For example, a special strain of rats, Eker rats, frequently suffers from a hereditary form of renal cell carcinoma. This cancer develops through multiple stages from early preneoplastic lesions, where renal tubules are morphologically altered, to the final cancer. Obviously a specific gene on the rat's chromosome 10, tsc2, is involved in the etiology of this cancer. In order to investigate this, phenotypically altered renal tubules as the earliest visible lesions were microdissected out of freeze-dried, 10-μm-thick tissue sections, with a focused dye laser (Kubo et al., 1995). The tubules were immediately placed in microvessels (Eppendorf tubes). With PCR and a suitable pair of primers it was tested to see whether the tsc2 gene is present in two versions (as expected for healthy cells) or if one version is lost, i.e. the tubules were tested for loss of heterozygosity (LOH). In fact, in approximately 20% of the tubules, LOH was detected in this very early stage of the cancer, indicating that LOH of tsc2 may be one of a number of causative changes in the etiology of this cancer.

In a second type of experiment, tissue sections of early gastric tumors were investigated by – PCR with respect to modifications in the cadherin E gene which codes for a cell adhesion protein (Becker et al., 1996, Schütze et al., 1997 a, b). Tissue sections of past cases were used in this retrospective study. It could be shown that, on the one hand, the laser treatment did not cause mutations in the cadherin gene. On the other hand, a point mutation was detected in a significant number of tumor cells which appears to be correlated with the progress of early gastric cancer.

## Selected Literature

I. Becker, K.F. Becker, M. Röhrl, G. Minkus, K. Schütze and H. Höfler (1996) Single cell mutation analysis of tumors from stained histologic slides. Lab. Investigations 75.6, 801–807.

P.J.H. Bronkhorst, G.J. Streekers, J. Grimbergen, E. Nijhof, J.J. Sixma and G.J. Brakenhoff (1995) A new method to study shape recovery of red blood cells using multiple optical trapping. Bioph. J. 69.5, 1666–1673.

P.J.H. Bronkhorst, J. Grimbergen, G.J. Brakenhoff, R.M. Heethaar and J. J. Sixma (1997) The mechanism of red cell disaggregation investigated by means of direct cell manipulation using multiple optical trapping. Brit. J. Hematol. 96, 256–258.

M.R. Emmert-Buck, R.F. Bonner, P.D. Smith, R.F. Chuaqui, Z. Zhuang, S.R. Goldstein, R.A. Weiss and L.A. Liotta (1996) Laser capture microdissection. Science 274, 998–1001.

Y. Kubo, F. Klimek, Y. Kikuchi, P. Bannasch and O. Hino (1995) Early detection of Knudson's two hits in pre-neoplastic renal cells of the Eker rat model by the laser microdissection procedure. Cancer Res. 55, 989–990.

W. Meier-Ruge, W. Bielser, E. Remy, F. Hillenkamp, R. Nitsche and E. Unsöld (1976) The laser in the Lowry technique for microdissection of freeze-dried tissue slices. Histoch. J. 8, 387–401.

K. Schütze, I. Becker, K.F. Becker, S. Thalhammer, R. Stark, W.M. Heckl, M. Böhm and H. Pösl (1997a) Cut out or poke in – the key to the world of single genes: laser micromanipulation as a valuable tool on the look-out for the origin of disease. Genetic Analysis 14, 1–8.

K. Schütze, M. Böhm, S. Thalhammer, R. Stark, W.M. Heckl, H. Pösl (1997b) Laser microbalation for genetic analysis on a single cell basis (in German). BIOforum 20, 82-87.

K. Schütze, G. Lahr (1998) Identification of expressed genes by laser mediated manipulation of single cells. Nature Biotechnology 16.8, 737–747.

K. Svoboda, C.F. Schmidt, D. Brante, S.M. Block (1992) Conformation and elasticity of the isolated red blood cell membrane skeleton. Bioph. J. 63, 784–793.

## 6.5 Laser microbeam and optical tweezers in reproduction medicine

Most problems of human infertility are caused organically and cannot be alleviated. In a high percentage of cases, however, the problems can be overcome by simply performing the process of sperm-egg fusion extracorporally in a reaction tube (*in vitro* fertilization, IVF). Often, an almost trivial mechanical problem is the cause of infertility: The mammalian egg is surrounded by a highly viscous envelope, the zona pellucida which cannot be penetrated by the sperm cells. Infertility is the consequence. This by no means influences the health of potential progeny; it is a purely mechanical problem.

One way to overcome the barrier is to aspire whole sperm cells in a glass capillary and to directly microinject by penetrating the zona pellucida micromechanically and injecting the sperm cell into the cytoplasma of the egg cell. This technique is called "intra cytoplasmic sperm injection", ICSI. Somewhat less intensive is "subzonal insemination" or SUZI. Here the zona pellucida, but not the egg cell membrane, is penetrated and the sperm is injected in the layer between zona and membrane. The last barrier, the egg cell's membrane is penetrated by the cell in the natural way, the way it would be after a sperm cell overcame the zona by own means. Experiments using laser microbeams provide basic insights into the processes underlying *in vitro* fertilization and have the prospect of becoming a useful tool for this technique. A large number of experimental approaches have already been published. Some typical examples will be reported below.

Occasionally a second problem can cause infertility: The motility of a sperm cell may be too low. Highly motile sperm cells are often said to be "high quality sperm" though it is not clear how motility of sperm should affect the health of progeny. In this sense the term high quality has to be seen strictly as a terminus technicus. The disadvantage of low motility may be overcome by the help of optical tweezers. Thus it is interesting to get quantitative information on sperm cell motility and on factors influencing it. Optical tweezers are well suited for such motility studies.

## 6.5.1 Laser zona drilling (LZD) and handling of sperm cells by optical tweezers

By drilling a micrometer sized hole in the zona pellucida, the viscuous barrier can be opened. Sperm cells approaching a thus-treated egg cell by chance will be attracted and can slip through the hole into its interior, where the normal processes of fertilization continue. In order to increase the chance of finding the channel through the zona, the sperm may be caught by the optical trap/optical tweezers and led to the entrance of the channel. Recent laser techniques combine zona drilling by a laser microbeam with optical trapping of sperm cells. It is a non-contact method in the sense that no micromechanical tools are required. Fig. 50 (from Schütze et al., 1995 and Clement-Sengewald et al., 1996) shows the principle.

In a model experiment with mouse gametes *in vitro* fertilization without laser support (IVF), laser zona drilling (LZD) and subzonal insemination (SUZI) assisted by optical tweezers were compared for efficiency (Enginsu et al., 1995). Two cases were investigated: normal insemination conditions, with 2 million sperm cells per ml and low insemination conditions with about a quarter of that cell density.

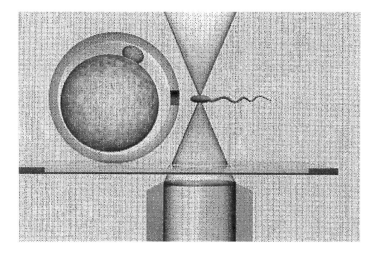

**Fig. 50:** *Schematic representation of laser zona drilling and laser capture of sperm: Using the microbeam a hole is drilled into the zona pellucida. Subsequently the sperm cell is captured with the optical tweezers and transported to the hole in the zona.*

Using a fifty to sixty 4 µJ pulses (337 nm) of 3 ns duration, a straight channel could be driven into the zona pellucida. For this operation, the egg cell did not have to be fixed by a micromanipulator, i.e., it was essentially a suspension procedure. An insemination was judged to be successful when the egg cell divided. Box 88 summarizes the major results of this study.

**Box 88: Success rates in mouse gametes of different types of fertilization techniques**

| Technique | Sperm density | Cells treated | Successfully fertilized | % success |
|---|---|---|---|---|
| Non laser IVF | normal | 85 | 45 | 53 |
| Laser zona drilling | normal | 124 | 74 | 60 |
| Non laser IVF | low | 63 | 21 | 33 |
| Laser zona drilling | low | 40 | 23 | 58 |
| Subzonal insemin. | low | 22 | 4 | 18 |

At high sperm density, there is not significant difference between conventional IVF and laser zona drilling technique. However, at low sperm density, the effect is significant with a 58% success rate with the laser supported technique as compared to 33% for the non laser technique. The very low success rate (18%) of subzonal insemination is not explained.

In conclusion, laser zona drilling appears to improve the success rates particularly at low sperm densities. What about optical tweezers? Do they provide an additional advantage? This question has been addressed in an experiment with bovine egg cells. (Clement-Sengewald et al., 1996). The overall result was that laser techniques alone (i.e. without any complementation of other techniques such as SUZI or IC-SY) yield successful fertilization, and the additional use of optical tweezers provides a small though significant increase in fertilization probability. Thus, the following basic studies on the effect of tweezer lasers on cell biological aspects of egg cells are of some practical importance.

## 6.5.2 Measuring effects of optical tweezers on sperm motility

A question of high importance is whether laser treatment induces damage to sperm. The major difficulty is to assess what is damage. Damage negligible in biophysical terms may be dramatic in terms of genetics. On the other hand, any technique of *in vitro* fertilization represents a tough treatment of germline cells, and damage based on such a treatment can only be assessed on the basis of long-term experience.

What can be assessed experimentally is the influence of laser irradiation on certain biophysical parameters. Examples are

- motility,
- linear velocity,
- actual distance traveled,
- maximum lateral head displacement, and
- motility patterns.

In addition, membrane permeability can be taken as criterion (see below). For the motility tests, a sperm cell can be held by optical tweezers for a given time and one can investigate the influence of laser treatment on the velocity of the sperm, which in turn is a measure for the damage induced by laser light. Box 89 summarizes the results of such an experiment.

Obviously there is no adverse effect on the velocity of the sperm after trapping for approximately 1 min with a 1 Watt NdYAG laser. When the duration of trapping exceeds a few minutes even at much smaller laser power (70 mW) damage can occur. This was checked with a continuous wave Ti Sapphire laser providing wavelengths of 760 nm and 800 nm (König et al., 1995). Human sperm cells were

**Box 89: Velocity before and after trapping a sperm cell with an NdYAG laser (output power 1W) for different times.**

| Exposure time | 15 sec | 45 sec | 120 sec |
|---|---|---|---|
| Motility before treatment | 19.6 | 22.5 | 24.2 |
| Motility after treatment | 23.5 | 24.7 | 16.2 |

stained with a live/dead fluorescence assay (Molecular probes). This assay uses two dyes, SYBR 14 (emission wavelength 515 nm, green) which penetrates the membranes of healthy cells, and propidium iodide (emission wavelength 636 nm, red) which can penetrate only the membranes of dead cells. Both dyes are excitable around 400 nm. Interestingly, the dyes can be excited with the Ti sapphire trapping laser due to two-photon effects (see Section 4.5). After trapping a sperm with 760 nm, for approximately 1 min, sperm cells originally fluorescing in green (live) change to red (dead). This color change does not occur during trapping by 800 nm for up to 10 min. Since the results were controlled by other live/dead distinguishing techniques (observation of flagellar rotation, assaying cloning efficiency), optical artifacts can be excluded. The basic result of this study is that 760 nm cause much higher damage than 800 nm. Whether this is due to an unknown absorption peak around 760 nm or reflects already the increased absorption of biological tissue in the visible range of the optical spectrum should be the subject of more detailed studies.

### 6.5.3 Laser inactivation of extra pronuclei

A regularly fertilized egg cell should contain two (pro) nuclei-carrying the genomes of the mother and the father. Since *in vitro* fertilization is often preceded by an intense hormone treatment, supernumerary male pronuclei occur in approximately 5% of all cases of IVF. All male pronuclei but one have to be removed for diploid regeneration, i.e. there is coexistence of two genomes – which is the standard for many organisms including mammals.

Laser experiments have been performed (Tadir et al., 1991) to remove supernumerary pronuclei by laser microirradiation and to study developmental effects of laser zona drilling (Schiewe et al., 1995).

This technique is probably not of practical importance for *in vitro* fertilization, since one can avoid transferring (re-implanting) fertilized egg cells with the incorrect number of pronuclei. However, the technique may be useful in basic research where, for example, the effects of hyperploidy in the early stage of development are studied, since triploidy of single human chromosomes, particularly that of chromosome 21, represents a massive health problem. Producing selected grades of ploidies by laser elimination of pronuclei may eventually have a significant practical aspect in studies on human genetics.

## 6.5.4 Helping childless couples: Do laser microtools improve human IVF?

Probably the most comprehensive use of lasers in the treatment of human infertility has been reported by Antinori et al., 1996. Two groups of patients have been treated by laser zona drilling for whom two to four non-laser IVF attempts had previously failed. This group of patients was compared with a group of 98 patients who received no laser support. Of 179 patients receiving laser zona drilling, 17 gave birth to healthy babies. Box 90 summarizes details.

**Box 90: Summary of details of the first large LZD-IVF treatment series**

| Laser treated | Group A | Group B | Group C |
|---|---|---|---|
| Number of patients | 107 | 72 | 98 |
| Mean maternal age | 38.1 yr | 38.2 yr | 37.8 yr |
| Previous IVF failures | 2–4 | | 2–4 |
| Laser treated embryos | 216 | 218 | 0 |
| Non laser treated embryos | 223 | 0 | 407 |
| Clinical pregnancies | 39 (36.4%) | 32 (44.4%) | 19 (19.3%) |
| Implantation rate per embryo | 9.3% | 16% | 5.1% |
| Normal babies born | 10 | 7 | 0 |
| Newborns per patient | 9.3% | 9.7% | 0 |

More than 1/3 of the patients who received laser treatment became pregnant; of the non-treated patients, less than 20% became pregnant. Birth was given only by women after laser treatment of the egg cells. Adding laser untreated embryos to the laser treated embryos did not improve the chance of pregnancy (group A versus group B). Thus, laser treatment is obviously the critical step in pregnancy induction.

These results are encouraging but the use of lasers in human IVF still has to be investigated in more detail before results are conclusive.

## 6.5.5 A word of caution

So far there is much enthusiasm over the success rates of all types of human IVF. Nevertheless, one should keep in mind that this is still purely basic research, in spite of the success story reported by the Antinori group. Thus, at present, laser-assisted fertilization still lies mainly in the realm of veterinary medicine where a purely experimental character is ethically acceptable. With regard to human therapy, some words of caution should be said, not with the aim of criticizing the success of the laser techniques but with view to preventing disappointment. There is a report from the Tel Hashomer Hospital in Tel Aviv, Israel, on two cases of cancer in children (Toren et al., 1995). In this hospital 312 children have been born as a result of IVF. One case of hepatoblastoma and one case of clear cell carcinoma have been detected. Since in the general population the combined probability for the occurrence of these cancers is approximately 38 cases per million people the two cases out of 312 are seen by the authors of the report as a sign for caution, in spite of the fact that true statistics are not possible based only on two cases. The second caveat is related particularly to laser zona drilling: it is known from experiments on single cell electrophoresis that even one laser pulse of a few millijoules energy can cause a considerable amount of DNA strand breaks in an individual cell of the immune system (de With et al., 1994). If these primarily single-strand breaks also occur in gametes and develop into permanent damage, laser zona drilling might impose an additional problem.

## Summary and outlook

Laser supported *in vitro* fertilization increases the probability of a successful pregnancy and is already used clinically. A slight additional effect in animal fertilization has been observed when the optical tweezers are used to capture the sperm, but experience with the human system does not yet exist.

## Selected literature

S. Antinori, H.A. Selman, B. Caffa, C. Panchi, G.L. Dani, and C. Versaci (1996) Zona opening of human embryos using a non-contact UV laser for assisted hatching in patients with poor prognosis of pregnancy. Hum. Reprod. 11.11, 2488–2492.

A. Clement-Sengewald, K. Schütze, A. Ashkin, G.A. Palma, G. Kerlen and G. Brem (1996) Fertilization of bovine oocytes induced solely with combined laser microbeam and optical tweezers. J. of Assisted Reproduction and Genetics 13.3, 259–265.

M.E. Enginsu, K. Schütze, S. Bellanca, M. Pensis, R. Campo, S. Bassil, J. Donnez and S. Gordts (1995) Micromanipulation of mouse gametes with laser microbeam and optical tweezers. Human Reproduction 10, 1761–1764.

K. König, H. Liang, M.W. Berns, B.J. Tromberg (1995) Cell damage by near-IR microbeams. Nature 377, 20-21.

M.C. Schiewe, J. Neev, N.I. Hazeleger, J.P. Balmaceda, M.W. Berns and Y. Tadir (1995) Developmental competence of mouse embryos following zona drilling using a non-contact holmium:yttrium scandium gallium garnet (Ho:YSGG) laser system. Human Reproduction 10, 1821–1824.

K. Schütze, A. Clement-Sengewald, F.D. Berg, G. Brehm and R. Schütze (1995) Videofilm: Laser microbeam and optical tweezers: Micromanipulation of gametes and embryos. Institute for the Scientific Film, Göttingen, Germany

Y. Tadir, W.H. Wright, O. Vafa, L.H. Liaw, R. Asch and M.W. Berns (1991) Micromanipulation of gametes using laser microbeams. Human Reproduction 6, 1011–1016.

A. Toren, N. Sharon, M. Mandel, Y. Neumann, G. Kenet, C. Kaplinski, J. Dor and G. Rechavi (1995) Cancer, 76, 2372–2374.

A. de With, G. Leitz and K.O. Greulich (1994) Excessive UV B laser induced DNA damage in lymphocytes observed by single cell gel electrophoresis following the comet assay. J. Photochem. Photobiol., 24.1, 47–53.

# 7 Appendix

While reading this book you may have occasionally wished for a somewhat more detailed explanation of the optics underlying the discussions of laser microbeams and optical tweezers. Unfortunately, even basic optics requires some extended knowledge of geometry and mathematics. This appendix tries to compile textbook knowledge and data from handbooks necessary for those who want to understand the optics of laser microtools in greater detail.

If you want to construct your own optical elements or at least to understand them in depth, you will need some information on properties of the materials you intend to use for the construction of your microtools. You may look all this up in other books – but you will need several of them. The purpose of the appendix is to reduce this mountain of books on optics or material constants which you would need to have on your desk when building laser microtools. The appendix should help you as a reference of first resort.

## A1 Geometrical optics

### A1.1 From waves to rays

At a sufficiently large distance, the light emitted by a classical light source can be described as a spherical wave. At an even larger distance from the light source, the sphere is large and the surface can be approximated by a plane, much in the way that, in everyday life, the surface of the spherical Earth is perceived as a plane. In other words, the light can be described as a plane wave. Once it is accepted that the wave is a plane it can be described by a vector perpendicular to its surface. The trajectory of it is a straight line, a ray, which perfectly describes the motion of the plane wave. That is the basis of geometrical optics: Such an approximation only works when all optical elements are much larger than the wavelength of the light.

## A1.2 Refraction and reflection

Thus, in vacuum and in any other homogeneous medium light propagates along a straight line. This is no longer the case at the surface between two media. The simplest case is that when light first travels in vacuum (air is a reasonable model) and then falls onto a thick slab of glass. When it impinges perpendicularly onto the surface, no change in direction occurs. When there is an angle $\alpha_1$ (the angle of incidence) relative to the direction perpendicular to the slab (the surface normal), it changes its direction (it is refracted). Its new direction is described by a new angle, $\alpha_2$, with respect to the surface normal (the angle of refraction). How much the angles of incidence and refraction differ depends on a material constant of the glass, its refractive index n. It is defined by

$$n = \sin \alpha_2/\sin \alpha_1 \quad (A1)$$

This definition is a simplified form of the Snell's Law

$$n_2/n_1 = \sin \alpha_1/\sin \alpha_2 \quad (A2)$$

which is valid for any two types of transparent media. The simpler equation A1 is a special case of equation A2 using $n_1=1$ for vacuum or air and setting $n_2=n$.

In real optics there are no infinite glass blocks but glass slabs of a given thickness. When the ray, after having been refracted at the front surface, falls onto the rear surface it is refracted a second time, now just by $-\alpha_2$, i.e. it has its original direction but is shifted spatially by a distance depending on the refractive index and the thickness of the glass slab.

There is an angle $\gamma$, for which $\alpha_2$ becomes 90° and thus $\sin \alpha_2=1$. The refracted ray then has the direction of the surface, i.e. it does not really enter the glass block. The ray is just at the transition from being refracted and reflected. Equation A1 then becomes

$$\sin \gamma = n_2/n_1 \quad (A3)$$

with $\gamma$ called the "glancing angle". Rays impinging under this or larger angles onto the glass surface cannot enter the glass block. Equation A3 is still valid, but now the ray remains in the same medium, i.e. $n_1=n_2$. It follows immediately that

$$\alpha_1 = \alpha_2 \quad (A4)$$

which is a simple but very basic law of reflection. In principle it follows from the fact that the velocity of light does not change by reflection. Fig. A1 gives a corresponding graphical representation.

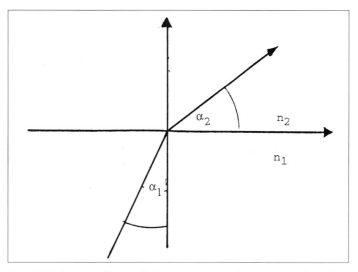

**Fig. A1:** *Refraction of a ray of light: It impinges with an angle α1 from the medium with the refractive index $n_1$ onto the surface between both media. When $n_2 > n_1$ the angle with respect to the surface normal is increased, i.e. a2 > a1. At some angle the refracted ray no longer enters the medium with refractive index $n_2$.*

## A1.3 Refraction by a spherical surface

While refraction by a glass slab is not of much practical value, refraction by a spherical surface is one of the most important processes of optics. It is the basis for almost any type of optical imaging. What does it mean when light falls parallel onto the optical axis on a spherical surface? Each partial ray sees only a very small fraction of the sphere. As it was discussed above, such a fraction is locally perceived as a plane. A beam on the optical axis senses a plane perpendicular to it, since the tangent of the spherical surface is perpendicular to the optical axis in that point. Thus a partial ray on the optical axis behaves as if it were to fall on a block of glass. It is not refracted.

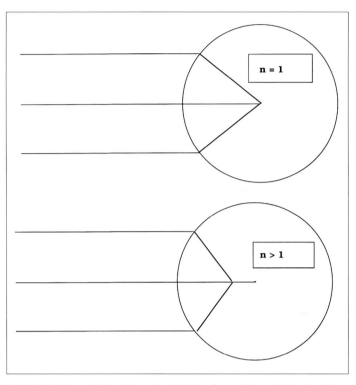

**Fig. A2:** *Light parallel to the optical axis is refracted by a spherical surface and collected into the center of the sphere. Since the index of refraction of the sphere is >1, the focal point is not identical with the sphere's center.*

But what happens to a partial ray that is parallel, but at a distance from the optical axis? There the tangent on the surface has a certain angle with respect to the optical axis. The partial ray, in spite of traveling parallel to the optical axis of the whole system, has an angle of incidence different from zero against the partial surface on which it impinges. A two-dimensional projection shows this angle.

In the unrealistic case where $\alpha_1$ and $\alpha_2$ are equal, it can be seen immediately that the partial ray would be refracted onto the radius of the sphere, i.e. it would finally pass through the sphere's center. This would happen to any partial ray falling on any point of the sphere, i.e. the whole incoming light would be focused in the sphere's center.

A real glass sphere has a larger refractive index than air. Here one can use one basic law of optics:

*an index of refraction n>1 merely shortens real distances by a factor of n. The optical path, the product of the real path with n, remains unchanged.*

The consequence of this law is that the construction of Fig. A2 is also valid in high refractive index, with the only exception that the point where all rays meet is no longer the geometrical center of the sphere but a point closer to the surface. This is the principle of focusing light by lenses.

## A1.4 The index of refraction for selected materials

The index of refraction for different transparent materials may vary by a factor of almost 2.5. The index of refraction of vacuum is 1, most gases are good models for vacuum. Glass may have an index of refraction from below 1.5 to almost 2 and diamond has a value of 2.4. The index of refraction for selected liquids (for example, the oil of the Cedar) may be higher than that of transparent solids (for example some glass, Box A1).

The index of refraction is related to the speed of light in a given medium, i.e. it has a much wider meaning than just being a material constant. In any medium with refractive index n the velocity of light can be calculated as

$$v = c/n. \quad (A5)$$

**Box A1: Index of refraction for different materials**

| | |
|---|---|
| Vacuum | 1.000 |
| Air 0 °C, 1 atm | 1.00029317 |
| Water | 1.3345 |
| Oil of the Cedar | 1.5180 |
| Quartz glass | 1.4601 |
| Plexiglas (PMMA) | 1.4931 |
| Flint glass SF 59 | 1.76167 |
| Boron glass BK1 | 1.51201 |
| Diamond | 2.4235 |

The theory of relativity states that no velocity faster than c is possible. Thus, refractive indices of all materials must have a value equal to or larger than 1, otherwise v would exceed c. In fact, all refractive indices given above are larger than 1. Particularly, the velocity of light in diamond is only of the order of $1.24 \cdot 10^{10}$ cm/s. Since $c = \lambda \cdot v$, either $\lambda$ or $v$ or both quantitites may be reduced in media with high refractive index. It turns out that it is the wavelength, but not the frequency which is reduced. In principle this can be expected from the fact that the energy of a light quantum $E = h \cdot v$ should not change when a light quantum enters a medium with higher refractive index.

## A1.5 Wavelength dependence on the index of refraction

**Box A2: Index of refraction for Suprasil Quartzglass (Heraeus, Hanau, FRG), water and flint glass for laser wavelengths used in laser microtools**

| Wavelength (nm) | Laser | n (quartz) | n water | n flint glass |
|---|---|---|---|---|
| 266 | NdYAG·4 | 1.500 | | |
| 308 | XeCl excimer | 1.486 | | |
| 337 | nitrogen | 1.479 | | |
| 355 | NdYAG·2 | 1.476 | | |
| 435.8 | | | | |
| 488 | Argon ion | 1.463 | | |
| 514.5 | Argon ion | 1.462 | | |
| 532 | NdYAG·2 | 1.461 | | |
| 694.3 | ruby | 1.455 | 1.340 | 1.642 |
| 768.2 | | | 1.329 | 1.610 |
| 905 | GaAs, Ti Sapphire | 1.452 | | |
| 1064 | NdYAG | 1.450 | | |

The index of refraction is wavelength-dependent. In the visible spectrum the effect is in the range of one percent – not much, but sufficient to cause several problems in optical imaging. For most practical purposes it is sufficient to know the index for a number of selected wavelengths and to interpolate linearly when the index for a wavelength between two known values is required. Today, with the availability of dye lasers, one might choose wavelengths in units of 50 or 100 nm. Historically other wavelengths have been chosen since they were available as emission lines of readily available substances such as the elements H, He, Na, K, or Hg. Box A2 lists the indices of refraction for a few materials relevant in optical imaging for different wavelengths. When it is a laser-typical wavelength, the name of the laser is indicated, too.

## A1.6 Reflection below the glancing angle

Even below the glancing angle, not all the light impinging on glass will be transmitted. At visible wavelengths and low intensity, a small fraction will be absorbed, but this is generally hardly recognizable. However, even below the glancing angle, some of the intensity is reflected. The degree of reflection is dependent on the angle of incidence.

At low angles (with good approximation up to $\alpha_1=50°$) the degree of reflection can be estimated by

$$r = (n'-n)^2/(n'+n)^2. \quad (A6)$$

For the interface between air (n=1) and boron glass (n'=1.51) one can calculate that a fraction of 0.041 (or 4.1%) is reflected. At an air/diamond (n'=2.42) interface this value is 17.1%. Thus the diamond appears to be bright as if it were a light source itself. This is one of the secrets of the beauty of a diamond. A second secret is that not only reflection, but also interference (see Appendix A4) and the generation of colors are governed by differences and ratios of the index of refraction.

In a glass slab of limited thickness light can be reflected at the front surface and at the rear surface. When one is looking through a window into daylight, reflection is hardly perceived. If one is looking from an illuminated room into the dark, however, the reflected light becomes dominant and one can see a mirror image of the interior of the room. Often, this is a double image, since there are reflections at both surfaces of the slab. Similarly as for the transmission through the slab as described above, the image reflected from the rear surface is slightly shifted so that the two images are slightly shifted with respect to each other.

Since part of the light reflected at the rear surface can be reflected a second time at the front surface and thus, after being slightly shifted, be transmitted through the slab, double images can also occur in transmission. The doubly reflected signal has an intensity of only 0.16%. Generally this causes no problems in normal life. In laser microscopy, however, where high light intensities are used, these signals can have considerable intensity and perturb experimental observations. Occasionally, in laser microbeams one can make use of this effect to generate a double microbeam with distinctly different intensities of the partial beams. In most cases, however, such reflections are unwanted and should be prevented by coating (see next section).

## A1.7 Coating of optical elements

**Box A3: Index of refraction at selected wavelengths of materials used for coating**

(Modified from H. Naumann, G. Schröder (1992) Bauelemente der Optik, Carl Hanser, München)

| Material | | n at (l) | |
|---|---|---|---|
| | | (l in mm) | Region of transparency |
| (mm) | | | |
| Kryolithe | $Na_3AlF_6$ | 1.35 (0.55) | 0.2–14 |
| Magnesium fluoride | $MgF_2$ | 1.38 (0.55) | 0.2–5 |
| Cerium fluoride | $CeF_3$ | 1.70 (0.6) | 0.3–5 |
| Thorium fluoride | $ThF_4$ | 1.52 (0.5) | 0.2–15 |
| Zinc sulfide | ZnS | 2.35 (0.6) | 0.4–14 |
| Aluminium oxide | $Al_2O_3$ | 1.63 (0.55) | 0.2–7 |
| Silicium dioxide | $SiO_2$ | 1.46 (0.55) | 0.2–8 |
| Silicium monoxide | SiO | 1.46 (0.55) | 0.6–7 |
| Titanium dioxide | $TiO_2$ | 2.61 (0.59) | 0.4–12 |
| Zirkonium oxide | $ZrO_2$ | 2.1 (0.55) | 0.3–7 |
| Silicium | Si | 3.46 (2) | 0.9–8 |
| Germanium | Ge | 4.0 (10) | 1.8–35 |
| Lead-telluride | PbTe | 4.1 (1) | 4–20 |

As equation A6 shows, the degree of reflection is primarily governed by the square of the difference of the indices of refraction. If, for example, at the air–glass interface discussed above, an additional layer of material with n=1.23 is introduced, the reflection at the air-layer interface is 1.06%, and that of the layer glass interface 1.04%. The total reflection is then approximately 2% instead of 4.1% at an air-glass interface. For such a simple system the minimal reflection is achieved when

$$n_{layer} = \sqrt{n \cdot n'}. \quad (A7)$$

Reflection is decreased even further when a gradient of refractive indices is built up, which is possible by modern thin layer technology. Then, reflection can be almost completely suppressed. Processes whereby such a layer is introduced are called "coating". Coating may be used to decrease, but also to increase reflectivity. Since the refractive index is a function of material and wavelength, coating conditions can be found which reduce the reflectivity of an optical element for certain wavelengths, or in other words: reflectivity can be wavelength-optimized. The materials which are used for coating have to form stable layers. For high power optical elements they have to be heat resistant and they have to be sufficiently transparent in order to prevent absorption. Box A3 lists some often used materials and their refractive indices.

## A1.8 Light guides: Simple optical instruments

Total reflection can be used to construct a very simple optical element, the light guide. It may either have the form of a slab or, more practically, a very thin long cylinder (a sort of wire). In the cylindrical form, a core with index of refraction $n_1$ (typically, a few up to a few hundred micrometers in diameter) is enveloped by a cladding with refractive index $n_2$. Light entering the light guide at angles smaller that the critical angle will be totally reflected until it leaves the light guide through its end surface. Fig. A3 shows the principle.

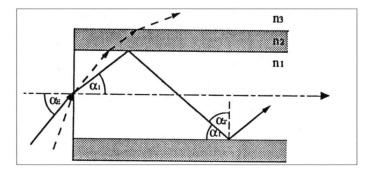

**Fig. A3:** *Transport of light through a light guide. The angle of acceptance can be calculated from the two refractive indices by Equation A7.*

## A1.9 Prisms

Apart from lenses, prisms are useful optical elements in microscopy and thus also in laser microtools. Prisms can be used to change the path of optical rays and they can be used to split white light in different colors.

Fig. A4 shows a simple prism. In the given example, the cross section is a triangle with one angle of 90 degrees and two angles of 45 degrees. A ray falling orthogonally onto one of the small surfaces enters the prism without being deflected. At the rear surface, which has an angle of 45 degrees with respect to the direction of the ray, the latter is deflected by 2·45=90 degrees and leaves the prism unperturbed via the second small surface. In principle the same change in direction could have been accomplished with a simple mirror, but prisms are much better suited in terms of transparency and stability of adjustment. Many other forms of prisms exist which may change a ray's direction in many different ways. Some of them invert an image, others keep it in upright position.

Prisms are also used to split white light into different colors. Here the ray falls on one surface at a given angle. Then it is deflected as shown in Fig. A4. Since, however, the index of refraction is wavelength-dependent, different colors are deflected in different ways. The colors leave the prism under different angles. When they are projected onto a screen, a beautiful rainbow-like image can be generated.

Another type of prism is the Wollastone prism which was used for calibration of optical tweezers (Section 2.6.5). It splits a beam of polarized light into two beams of perpendicularly polarized light (see also Appendix A4.3).

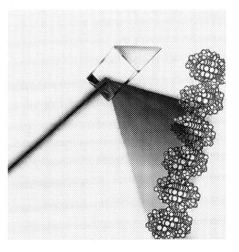

**Fig. A4:** *Splitting of white light into rainbow colors after passing through a prism.*

# A2 Ray optics: Lenses and image formation

## A2.1 Lenses

In Appendix A1.3 we saw that spherical surfaces can collect light. An optical element where one surface is part of a sphere is a lens. Even when a lens is fully illuminated by parallel light, the angle of incidence is different at any point of the spherical surface. Geometrical considerations in the previous chapter have shown that in this case all partial rays are refracted towards one single point, the focus (see Fig A5) The distance of the focus from the lens, the focal length, can be calculated from the radius of the spherical surface and the refractive index of the material used:

$$1/f = n \cdot 1/r. \quad (A8)$$

This is only correct for (theoretically) thin lenses. A realistic lens has a second surface at its rear part. Quite often this is also spherical, albeit with another radius. Then

$$1/f = n/r_1 + n/r_2. \quad (A9)$$

When the index of refraction of the lens is large or when the radii of the surface spheres are small, then $\vee 1/f$ becomes large. Consequently the reciprocal, f, will be small.

Each lens, even asymmetric ones, has two foci equidistant from the center of the lens. This is not the case for systems of lenses (for example, objectives).

## A2.2 Different types of lenses

One single spherical surface makes a lens. Thus, the simplest lenses have one spherical and one flat surface. This may be convex or concave. Many lenses two have spherical surfaces in any combination. Thus we have
- · convex lenses
- · biconvex lenses,
- · concave lenses,
- · biconcave lenses, and
- · concave-convex lenses.

The concave lenses always generate virtual images and have, formally, negative focal lengths. In the following, primarily convex lenses are discussed.

## A2.3 Imaging by a simple lens

For imaging by a lens, the following rules apply:
1  Partial rays falling onto the lens parallel to the optical axis will go through the opposite focus (as already discussed above).
2  Partial rays going through one focus will leave the lens parallel (this is essentially rule 1 but in reverse).
3  Partial rays through the center of the lens are unaffected.

Figs A5 and A6 show how these rules help to construct the imaging by a lens.

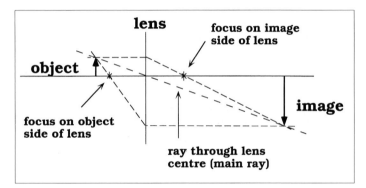

**Fig. A5:** *Focusing parallel light by a spherical lens.*

In order to get some idea about the imaging properties of a simple lens we analyze the imaging of an arrow with its base on the optical axis and its tip pointing perpendicular to it, i.e. an arrow pointing parallel to the lens. The tip of the arrow can be regarded as a point source of light. Many partial rays emerge from the tip. One of them impinges on the lens parallel to the optical axis, and according to rule 1, will go through the opposite focus. Another one goes through the focus on the side of the arrow. It will leave the lens parallel to it. The section point of the two partial rays is the image of the arrow's tip. As a control, we can analyze a third partial ray, the one going straight through the center of the lens. It has also to go through the image point.

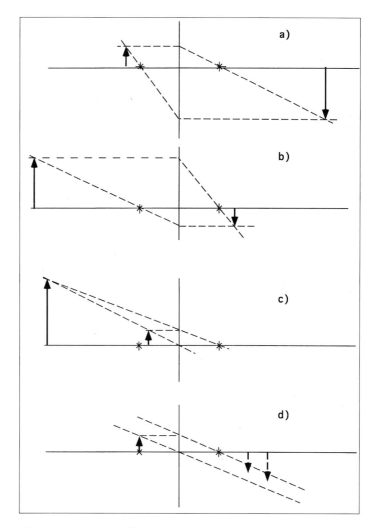

**Fig. A6:** *Construction of image formation by lenses under several geometric conditions.*

Fig. A6 a–d show such constructions for different positions of the arrow. The types of image are very different. When the arrow is located at distances further than the focal distance f, as in fig. A6 a and b, one can actually draw a corresponding arrow on the other side of the lens. This is a real image. It can be projected onto a screen. Alternatively it can be looked at with a second lens and thus become part of a telescope or microscope. When the arrow is exactly in the focus, we have a special case. Strictly, we cannot draw an arrow according to the rules given above, since the partial rays emanating from the tip of the arrow have no intersection. If we go far enough to the right, the image is large compared to the distance between the two parallel rays and every point of the arrow corresponds again to an approximate point of the image. This is the principle of a standard magnifying glass. The big advantage of this type of imaging is that we can pick the image up at any position on the right side of the lens. A totally different situation occurs when the arrow on the left side is closer than the focus. Then we cannot draw an image on the right side. However, we get some type of image on the left side. This is a virtual image. It can be looked at, but it cannot be projected onto a screen. Box A4 summarizes the results.

**Box A4: Type of image for different positions of the object with respect to the lens focus**

| Position of the arrow | Type of image | Size of image |
|---|---|---|
| Further away than 2 f | Real | Diminished in size |
| Between 2f and f | Real | Enlarged |
| Exactly at f | Infinite | Enlarged |
| Closer than f | Virtual | Enlarged |

It is also possible to give a quantitative value for the imaging ratio: An arrow with the size A will have an image size I given by

$$I/A = i/f \quad (A10)$$

where f is the focal length, as above, and i is the distance of the image from the lens. This can be verified in the constructions of Fig. A6.

## A2.4 Magnification and the thin lens equation

From Fig. A6 a–d one can see that imaging by a lens can be described by a simple geometric construction. This allows one to derive some simple equations which relate object size and distance, image size and distance and the focal length with each other.

The most simple relationship gives the magnification Magn achieved by the lens, which is defined as the height of the image, $h_{image}$ divided by the height of the object, $h_{object}$.

The dotted line in Fig. A6 a, connecting the tip of the object arrow with the tip of the image arrow, intersects the optical axis in the center of the lens under an angle $\alpha$. The tangents of this angle can be calculated in two ways:

$$\tan \alpha = h_{object}/s_{object} \quad or \quad \tan \alpha = h_{image}/s_{image}, \quad (A11)$$

where $s_{object}$ and $s_{image}$ are the distances of object and image from the lens. Combining the two one obtains

$$Magn = h_{image}/h_{object} = s_{image}/s_{object}. \quad (A12)$$

The magnification can be calculated in a second way, by shifting the object arrow into the plane of the lens and using the triangles formed by the dashed line in Fig A6a. With identical arguments the result is then

$$Magn = (s_{image}-f)/f. \quad (A13)$$

Combining Equation A12 and A13 gives

$$(s_{image}-f)/f = s_{image}/s_{object}. \quad (A14)$$

Resolving the bracket, dividing of the whole equation by $s_{image}$ and slight rearrangement finally gives the *Thin lens equation:*

$$1/f = 1/s_{image}+1/s_{object}. \quad (A15)$$

Caution: Since we have chosen a case where the image is real, no convention about plus and minus signs in the calculation were needed. With other types of lenses and imaging the following conventions are needed:

1  focal lengths of diverging lenses are negative,
2  distances of virtual images are negative, and
3  positive magnifications designate upside down images;
   negative magnifications designate upright images (in some textbooks the convention is vice versa).

After multiplication of the thin lens equation with f and with $s_{object}$ one obtains

$$s_{object} = (f/Magn)+f. \quad (A16)$$

For large magnifications the first term becomes small, i.e. $s_{object}$ is approximately the focal length f, in agreement with the geometrical constructions of Fig. A6 where the largest images were obtained with objects close to the focus.

## A2.5 The magnifying glass

The magnifying glass is the simplest optical instrument. It is the lens described in Fig. A6 a. The object is placed between lens and focus, i.e. a virtual image is generated and looked at by the human eye. Since the optimal reading distance of the human eye is approximately 25 cm, the magnifying glass ideally is held in a position which corresponds to an image distance of 25 cm. Since a virtual image is generated, for the calculation of the magnification by Equation A16 the negative value of -25 cm has to be taken for $s_{image}$:

$$Magn = (-25 \text{ cm-f})/f = -(1+25 \text{ cm/f}). \quad (A17)$$

For example, a lens with a focal length of 5 cm magnifies by a factor of 6. The negative value for the magnification indicates an upright image.

## A2.6 Aberrations, lens errors

A number of lens errors lead to aberrations in the optical imaging. The most important are spherical aberration and chromatic aberration.

Spherical aberration causes a point to be not exactly imaged as a point but as a disc with a finite radius. If the image is projected onto a screen, the type of image seen depends on the distance $d_{screen}$ and the image distance $s_{image}$ as defined above. Only when the screen is sufficiently far away from $s_{image}$ will the image be a disc with homogeneous intensity. In some positions it appears as a bright ring filled with lower intensity light, sometimes as a bright spot in a disc of lower intensity. When the screen is close to $s_{image}$ it looks like a bright spot with a ring (much like the planet Saturn observed from its poles) The reason for this aberration is that the lens has a certain thickness (thin lenses as discussed above do not really exist) and that it has a certain diameter. In some sense the parts of the lens close to the optical axis have a slightly longer focal length than the parts far away, i.e. at the edges of the lens. A graphical representatian of the partial ray along the optical axis is called a "caustic" representation.

Spherical aberration can be avoided by using an aperture of small diameter which allows the imaging only of partial rays close to the optical axis. The price for this improvement is the loss of brillance of the image. In most cases such a compromise is unacceptable. A much better way to avoid spherical aberration is to replace the single lens by a double lens made from glasses with different indices of refraction as shown in Fig A7.

While spherical aberration occurs also with monochromatic light, chromatic aberration is a problem of color imaging. Since the focal length of a lens depends on the refractive index of its material and the latter depends on the wavelength (see Section 3.5), the focal length is wavelength-dependent. Then similar imaging errors occur as for spherical aberration, but now the image of a white object becomes rainbow colored instead of structured in intensity, an effect which is often seen in cheap optical toys for children such as magnifying glasses made from plastics.

Again such a lens error can be corrected by a double lens similar to that shown in Fig. A7.

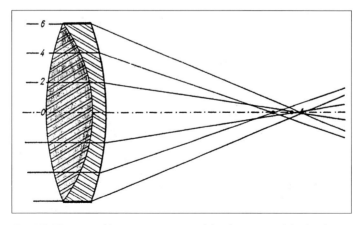

**Fig. A7:** *The second lens corrects some of the distortions of the first lens and in total the focal lengths of the partial rays become similar, as one would expect from an ideal lens. (From: K. Michel, Die Grundzüge der Theorie des Mikroskops, Wiss. Verlagsges. Stuttgart 1994.)*

## A2.7 The numerical aperture of a lens

One important parameter describing the quality of a lens is the amount of light which it can collect from an object in, or close to, the focus. This is equivalent to the requirement for an angle $\alpha$ being as large as possible, under which the lens is seen from the focus. A more detailed mathematical analysis reveals that it is not the angle itself, but its sine which describes a good lens. Unfortunately, the sine can never be larger than 1. However, in optics not the real paths, but the optical paths are relevant. As was already mentioned in Appendix A1, the optical path is obtained by multiplying the real path with the refractive index. Consequently, the quantity describing the quality of a lens is not $\sin \alpha$ but

$$A = n \cdot \sin \alpha. \quad (A18)$$

This is the numerical aperture. We have already learned in Section 1.3.6 and will see in Sections 4.3.2 and 4.3.3 that it determines the best focusing of a laser microbeam and optical tweezers as well as the resolution of a microscope. In principle, it can be made large when a transparent material with large refractive index is brought between lens and focus. In practical work, $\sin \alpha = 1$ is rarely reached and n does not exceed 1.6. Thus, numerical apertures of 1.4. are the present upper limit for commercially available microscope objectives (see Box 8 in Section 1.3.6).

# A3 Resolution of a microscope and focusing a laser

## A3.1 The Bessel function and maximal focusing of a laser

In Section A2 geometrical constructions were used to understand the imaging by lenses. There, in principle, it was possible to image an object onto a point in three dimensional space, i.e. into a sphere with radius zero. In real optics this is not possible, since it would result in an infinite power density in the focus. When the image size approaches the submicrometer range, diffraction will govern the imaging process and the wave nature of light has to be taken into account.

Optical elements confine this wave in space and this will cause diffraction. The diffraction effects can be calculated by mathematical equations called "differential equations". (Don't worry, we will not have to solve them.) Many optical elements are approximately cylindrical in shape (for example microscope objectives). For a cylindrical geometry the mathematical solutions of the differential equation are described by a family of mathematical functions called the Bessel functions. For the calculation of diffraction effects in a microscope comparatively simple sorts of Bessel function, those of first order, are relevant. Fig. A8 shows such a first order Bessel function.

It resembles a highly distorted sine function. Actually it can be expressed as a combination of sine and cosine functions. A detailed analytical calculation requires some mathematical effort. One can, however, derive the resolution of the microscope just by looking at the x values where the Bessel function is zero. This is the case at x values of 3.83, 7.01, 10.17.... The maxima and minima are at x values of 0, 5.13, 8.41, 11.61.... We will also be interested in the numerical values of the square of the Bessel function (see Box A5).

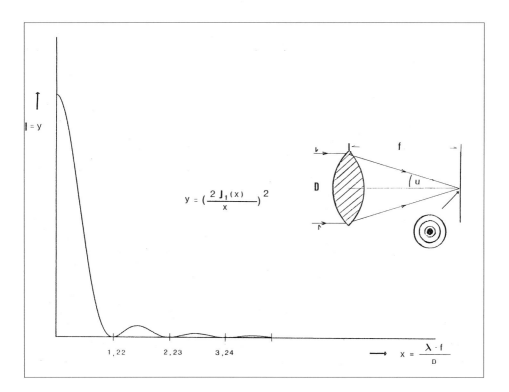

$$y = \left( \frac{2\, J_1(x)}{x} \right)^2$$

$$x = \frac{\lambda \cdot f}{D}$$

**Fig. A8:** Bessel function of first order.

**Box A5: Numerical values for the square of the first order Bessel function $J_1(x)$**

| x | 0 | 3.83 | 5.13 | 7.01 | 8.41 | 10.17 | 11.61 |
|---|---|------|------|------|------|-------|-------|
| 100·square (x) | 100 | 0 | 1.75 | 0 | 0.42 | 0 | 0.16 |

In order to convert this purely mathematical function into a function describing image formation in the microscope, one has to relate the variables J(x) and x with measurable quantities involved in imaging. A well measurable quantity describing the imaging process would be the radial light intensity distribution in the image (i.e. the intensity as a function of radial distance from the optical axis), for example, if a screen were located at some distance from the objective (in direction of light propagation). At this position the focal point would be enlarged by the factor R (see below).

The result of the mathematical analysis is that the intensity distribution can be calculated from the Bessel function when x is related to measurable quantities by the following equation

$$x = (2\pi \cdot r \cdot n \cdot \sin \alpha)/(\lambda \cdot R), \quad (A19)$$

thereby r is now the radial distance from the optical axis, $\lambda$ is the wavelength, n the refractive index in the light path, R is the ratio of image size to size in the focal plane (which will increase with increasing axial distance from the objective) and $\alpha$ is the half angle under which the objective is seen.

We know that J(x), square (x) and consequently the light intensity becomes zero when x is 3.83. We are now interested in for which value of r (which we will now call $r_0$) this is the case. The equation becomes now

$$3.83 = (2\pi \cdot r_0 \cdot n \cdot \sin \alpha)/(\lambda \cdot R) \quad (A20)$$

or after simple rearrangements and taking $3.83/2\pi = 0.61$

$$r_0 = (0.61 \cdot \lambda \cdot R)/(n \cdot \sin \alpha). \quad (A21)$$

At the distance $r_0$ a dark ring will appear on the screen. The smallest possible ring radius will be measured when the screen is moved into the focal plane where R=1 (that's how R was defined). The radius of the first dark ring around the central bright spot is then

$$r_{min} = (0.61 \cdot \lambda)/(n \cdot \sin \alpha) \quad (A22)$$

and the diameter is correspondingly

$$d_{min} = 1.22 \cdot \lambda / n \cdot \sin \alpha. \quad (A23)$$

The diameter $d_{min}$ is also called the diameter of the Airy disc. It is the central spot of the ring system containing 84% of the whole intensity. The first bright ring, beyond $d_{min}$ contains 7.2% and the second bright ring contains 2.8% of the total intensity. This intensity ratio may be shifted in favor of the rings at non-optimal focusing.

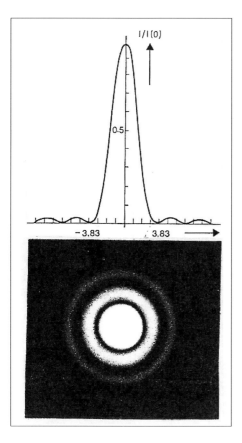

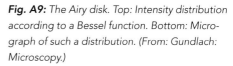

**Fig. A9:** The Airy disk. Top: Intensity distribution according to a Bessel function. Bottom: Micrograph of such a distribution. (From: Gundlach: Microscopy.)

$$A = n \cdot \sin \alpha \quad (A24)$$

the numerical aperture, has already been defined in Section A2.7. With it, the radius of the Airy disc in the focal plane becomes

$$d_{min} = 1.22 \cdot \lambda / A \quad (A25)$$

It is reasonable to use $d_{min}$ as the diameter of a focused light source, since a further size reduction is not possible. Since the largest available numerical apertures are close to 1.4, the minimal diameter of the Airy disc is only a function of the wavelength.

*The minimal available focus diameter ≈ 0.86·λ ≈ 7/8·λ.   (A26)*

## A3.2 The resolution of a microscope

The resolution of a microscope, i.e. the smallest distance at which two objects can still be seen separately, also follows immediately from the minimum for the Bessel function. When two objects are imaged by a microscope, both of them generate Airy discs with ring systems. The rings of one object may coincide with the Airy disc of the neighbor. Since, however, only a small percentage of light intensity is in the rings, this does not harm much. But when the two objects approach each other further, the Airy discs themselves begin to overlap. Good distinction is possible when one Airy disc falls just in the first minimum of the other. The quantity which is relevant is now the radius (not, as above, the diameter) of the Airy disc:

$$r_{min} = 0.61 \cdot \lambda / A. \quad (A27)$$

Strictly speaking, this is the shortest distance which may separate two point light sources which are still to be observed as two sources. The resolution of a microscope is somewhat different. In most cases objects are illuminated by an external light source. One can easily imagine that the quality of illumination contributes to resolution. A theory developed by Ernst Abbe showed that for illumination the numerical aperture also is relevant. The total resolution of the system is then

$$r_{min} = 1.22 \cdot \lambda (A_{objective} + A_{condenser}). \quad (A28)$$

This is the Abbe criterion for the complete resolution of a microscope. When the aperture of the condenser is as large as that of the objective the equation for the resolution of the point sources is obtained. Unfortunately, a large aperture provides poor contrast. Thus the numerical aperture of the condenser cannot be made too large. A good practical compromise is that it should be not larger than 2/3 of the numerical aperture of the objective. Thus the practical optimum for resolution (with an objective aperture of 1.4 and a condenser aperture of 0.93) can be expressed as:

$$Practical\ resolution \approx 0.86 \cdot \lambda \quad (A29)$$

which is identical to A26.


## A3.3 Experimental determination of focal radii

The ideal conditions assumed in the discussion above may not be present in a real microscope. Therefore, when the actual spot size is required, for example, in theoretical calculations of optical trapping forces, they have to be measured. One approach is to move, with submicrometer accuracy, a knife edge through the beam and measure the intensity still reaching a detector behind the object plane. Since with a knife edge it is difficult to find the first diffraction minimum, one measures the radial distance from 90% maximal intensity to 10% maximal intensity. The spot radius obtained by this approach is in principle smaller than the diameter of the Airy disc.

It is approximately

$$r_{90\%-10\%} = \lambda/(\pi \cdot \theta), \quad (A30)$$

where $\theta$ is the half focusing angle which can be calculated from the numerical aperture. The experimental result for a NdYAG laser ($\lambda$=1064 nm) and different 100x objectives (all Zeiss objectives) is summarized in Box A6 (adapted from Wright et al., 1994).

For the two objectives with a numerical aperture of 1.3 the spot radii differ by 13%. In turn, the radii for the same objective having the aperture set to 1.25 and to 1.00, the spot radii are almost identical. This underlines the necessity of experimental determination of focusing parameters.

**Box A6: Experimental determination of spot radii $r_{90\%-10\%}$ for three different 100x Zeiss objectives and five different apertures**

| Objective | Num. aperture | Spot radius (nm) |
|---|---|---|
| Neofluar | 1.3 | 390 |
| Neofluar for phase contrast | 1.3 | 440 |
| Plan variable num apert. | 1.25 | 540 |
| Plan variable num apert. | 1.00 | 530 |
| Plan variable num apert. | 0.80 | 610 |

## A3.4 Visibility of objects

**Box A7: Detectability for different qualities of illumination and different types of objects. In the original work (Francon, 1966) the illumination conditions were termed as coherent, partially coherent and non-coherent.**

| Illumination | Coherent | Partial | Noncoherent |
|---|---|---|---|
| Two bright points on black background | 1.63 | 1.22 | 1.22 |
| Smallest radius of a just visible black disk on light background | 0.08 | 0.08 | 0.12 |
| Bright disk on black background | | Depends on illumination | |
| Smallest width of a just-recognizable black line on bright background | 0.01 | 0.01 | 0.02 |
| Bright line on black background | | Depends on illumination | |

Often extreme resolution is not really required, objects just have to be made visible. For example, when single molecules have to be handled by laser microbeam and optical tweezers one does not really need an exact imaging. Structures as small as 2 nm can be visualized by the light microscope but appear thicker than they really are. The minimal size which can be made visible depends on a number of parameters and can be formally given by the same equation as for resolution:

$$r_{min} = \Xi \cdot (\lambda/A) \quad (A31)$$

where Ξ is a dimensionless number, which differs for different conditions. For the resolution of the microscope Ξ was 1.22 at low aperture and 0.61 for the theoretical case of maximum aperture of the condenser. The former case is non-coherent, the latter is coherent illumination. Box A7 lists some such values for a number of different conditions and different types of illumination.

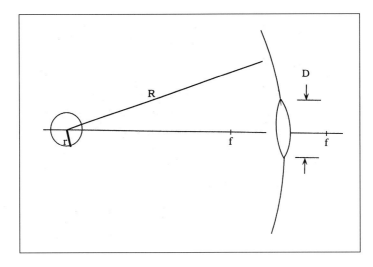

**Fig. A10:** *Geometry of light collection.*

## A3.5 Why lasers can be focused better than thermal light

So far, the discussion on focusing and resolution made one simplification which can be achieved only approximately in real microscopy: it assumed point light sources. A point source can be located in the focus of a lens or a spherical mirror will produce strictly parallel light. This in turn can be used to obtain an ideal focus. Unfortunately, in reality a point source can only be approximated by a small bulb and a large diameter lens or mirror. The light can be made reasonably parallel, but most of the light will finally be lost. Fig. A10 shows the geometry of light collection.

Real focusing means to project a real object, for example a bulb, into the focus so that its size is close to the wavelength of the light used. Because of diffraction, a geometry which theoretically would result in a smaller image is useless. In turn, a geometry which results in a larger image would not fully exploit the focusing power of the lens or the objective. With green light ($\lambda$=500 nm) and a bulb of radius B, the imaging equation of section 3.7 can be used to calculate the distance b, at which the bulb has to be positioned from the lens:

$$b = B \cdot (f/500) \text{ nm} \quad (A32)$$

When W is the power of the bulb, then its power density at a distance b, i.e. at the position of the lens, is

$$w = W/(4\pi \cdot b^2) \quad (A33)$$

When a lens or objective with a numerical aperture close to 1 (in air) is used, its radius is approximately its focal length, i.e. its cross section is

$$A = 4\pi \cdot f^2 \quad (A34)$$

and the power which is falling on the lens is

$$W' = w \cdot A = (4\pi \cdot f^2 \cdot W)/(4\pi \cdot b^2) \quad (A35)$$

$$W' = (W \cdot f^2)/b^2 \quad (A36)$$

f/b is just the size reduction R. Thus one obtains

$$W' = W \cdot R^2. \quad (A37)$$

Here we see the dilemma: we can get a size reduction, i.e. come close to ideal focusing, but the loss in power goes with the square of R.

What we have discussed here may appear too pessimistic to those readers who know how a spot light or the front lights of a car work. There, a point source – the bulb – is located in the focus of a mirror and approximately parallel light is generated. But the quality of the parallel light is better when the ratio between mirror diameter to bulb diameter is large. This, however, means that power density of the bulb is "diluted". The mathematical problem is equivalent to that described above, even the same formula holds.

In conclusion, only lasers have a sufficiently small divergence $\Theta$ to obtain high power densities in the focus.

## Selected literature

M. Francon and G. Braun (1966) Introduction in new methods of light microscopy. Karlsruhe FRG.

H. Gundlach (1994) Microscopy in: Ullmanns Encyclopedia of Industrial Chemistry, VCH Weinheim, FRG.

W.H. Wright, G.J. Sonek and M.W. Berns (1994) Parametric study of the forces on microspheres held by optical tweezers. Applied Optics 33, 1735–1748.

# A4 Light as a wave: Mathematical representation

## A4.1 The wave equations

In this chapter the basic mathematical tools are collected which will allow us to describe interference, polarization and standing light waves.

Unlike, for example, water waves, electromagnetic waves do not require a medium. They can well travel in vacuum. Due to a coordinated interplay of the electric and the magnetic component of the electromagnetic field, the waves are self driving. The reason for this is that magnetic fields changing in time produce electric fields and vice versa.

Let us start with a situation where the amplitude of the electric component of the field begins to increase. It will reach a maximum value and then start to collapse. This change drives the increase of the magnetic component of the field which receives all the energy originally contained in the electric field. Then the magnetic field is maximal, starts to collapse and thus regenerates the electric field. For visible light, the cycle time is of the order of half a femtosecond ($10^{-15}$ sec), i.e. the frequency is of the order of $2 \cdot 10^{15}$ cycles per second. The wavelength is of the order of 0.5 μm, as was already stated in Section 1.1.1.

Since the interplay between electric and magnetic field is completely symmetric, it is sufficient to use either the electric or the magnetic field for a mathematical description of electromagnetic waves.

For a mathematical description of any wave, one can ask different questions. Two simple problems can be formulated in analogy to water waves:

1 Assume a boat is anchored at sea. One may want to describe how it bobs up and down with time, when the water is wavy. It is the simplest description of a wave.

2   Another simple question asks how, for example, a wave maximum moves towards the coast. This may be interesting for a surfer, who wants to pick up this wave maximum and to ride on it toward the beach.

Mathematical functions whose graphical representations resemble waves are the sine or the cosine functions. The argument of them may be an angle or a real number. Box A8 gives some numerical values.

**Box A8: Numerical values of the cosine function and the sine function**

| Angle in degrees | | 0 | 30 | 45 | 60 | 90 | 135 | 180 | 225 | 270 | 315 | 360 |
|---|---|---|---|---|---|---|---|---|---|---|---|---|
| Angle as real number | 0 | 0.52 | 0.79 | 1.05 | 1.57 | 2.35 | 3.14 | 3.92 | 0.75 | 5.50 | 6.28 |
| cos x | | | 1 | 0.87 | 0.71 | 0.5 | 0 | -0.71 | -1 | -0.71 | 0 | 0.71 | 1 |
| sin x | | | 0 | 0.50 | 0.71 | 0.87 | 1 | 0.71 | 0 | -0.71 | -1 | -0.71 | 0 |

The full cycle corresponds to 360° or 6.28 ($2\pi$). The sine and the cosine functions are shifted by 90°. This is their phase difference. At small values of the real number argument (up to approx. 0.5) of the sine function is approximately equal to its argument. Similarly, for small values of x the cosine function of (1.57-x) is approximately equal to x.

In the anchored boat analogy one is interested in the momentary amplitude of the wave with frequency $v$ as a function of time t. It can be can be described by

$$A(t) = A_0 \cdot \sin (2\pi \cdot v \cdot t) \quad (A38)$$

where $v$ is the frequency, t is the running time, $A_0$ is the maximum amplitude, corresponding to the highest deviation from the average height in the anchoring boat analogy. A is the amplitude at time t. This form of the wave equation can be used, for example, to describe how an atom or a molecule which is fixed in position senses the electric component of an electromagnetic field. Since the sine takes values from -1 to +1, amplitudes from $-A_0$ to $+A_0$ result from equation A38. In this formulation the average height would be zero (sea level without waves). Simple as it is, Equation A38 bears an interesting result: one can measure the frequency by just looking at the time course. In the boat example this can be measured by just determining the time from one maximum to the next – without looking through the windows. The reason for this is that the frequency $v$ and the time t are, in a very special mathematical sense, complementary variables which may be calculated from each other by a mathematical operation called Fourier transform.

The surfer in analogy 2 has another problem. In order to orient himself with respect to the wave – for example, to find out if he is just before of after a wave maximum, he has to take a snapshot of the wave. The amplitude is related to the position by

$$A(x) = A_o \cdot \sin (2\pi \cdot x/\lambda). \quad (A39)$$

In this case x has to be measured from a wave maximum.

The complete description of a wave in space and in time is then given by a suitable combination of Equations A38 and A39:

$$A(x,t) = A_o \cdot (\sin 2\pi) \cdot (x/\lambda - v \cdot t) \quad (A40)$$

## A4.2 Polarized light

A water wave, as was chosen to make the wave equations plausible, is a quite special wave. Since Earth's gravity is involved in the formation of water waves, their variation of amplitude can be described as an up and down movement, and this is perpendicular to the direction of motion (towards the shore) in a very defined way. Such a wave with only one spatial direction is called "transversally polarized". Direction in electromagnetic fields and thus also light waves is not determined *a priori*. Any oscillation in the y–z plane is possible. Then the mathematical description becomes difficult. However, there are experimental tools to generate polarized light, i.e. an electromagnetic wave defined equally well as a water wave. When light is sent through a suitable material it will induce the electrons of the material to oscillate. The electrons behave like antenna, i.e. they absorb the energy and re-emit it again. The electrons of polarizing materials can oscillate (almost) only in one direction. Consequently, the radiation oscillates in a defined direction in space – it is polarized. Thin films of a number of materials are good polarizers. Many sunglasses transmit only polarized light to the eyes since one has found that sunlight is partially polarized and use of polarized sunglasses intensifies perceived contrasts.

When polarized light is observed with a second polarizer (which is then called an analyzer) two extremes are possible. When the polarization direction of the analyzer is aligned exactly in the direction of the light polarization, all light will pass through. When the both directions are perpendicular, no light will pass through. One can easily test this by looking through two polarizing sunglasses and rotating them against each other. The intensity of the light reaching the eye will vary from a maximum to zero.

When two perpendicularly polarized waves of equal intensity which have a phase shift of 90 degrees are recombined, another type of polarization results: the electric field vector rotates around the line of light propagation. It is circularly polarized. When the intensities of the two component waves are not exactly equal, the polarization is elliptical. This ellipticity can be measured with high accuracy.

Transversal polarization has been used, for example, in the experiments described in Box 27 of Section 2.5.1. In the interferometers used for calibration of optical tweezers a pair of waves with exactly perpendicular polarization is generated by a "Wollastone" prism (see also Appendix A1.9). After having passed a precisely positioned sample, for example a microbead, they recombine to give a circularly polarized wave, when the object is exactly on the optical axis. When the bead is displaced by a fraction of a nanometer, the polarization becomes elliptical and from this ellipticity the exact position of the bead can be determined.

## A4.3 Interference

By a suitable system of mirrors two polarized waves can be overlayed; they will then travel simultaneously in space. The amplitudes of such waves add up. The result of such an addition is not trivial, it has to be calculated carefully. For simplicity we will assume that both waves have the same amplitude $A_0$:

One of the waves can be described by Equation A41

$$A(x,t) = A_0 \cdot (\sin 2\pi) \cdot (x/\lambda - v \cdot t). \quad (A41)$$

The second wave may be shifted (run behind the first) by distance $\delta$. It can then be described by

$$A(x,t) = A_0 \cdot (\sin 2\pi) \cdot (x/\lambda - n \cdot t + \delta). \quad (A42)$$

If they both add up one obtains

$$A_{sum}(x,t) = A_o \cdot (\sin 2\pi) \cdot (x/\lambda - v \cdot t) + A_o \cdot (\sin 2\pi) \cdot (x/\lambda - n \cdot t + \delta). \quad (A43)$$

In order to add the two sine functions with different arguments we have to use a formula from trigonometrics:

$$(\sin a) + (\sin b) = 2 \cdot (\sin (a+b)/2 \cdot \cos (a-b)/2. \quad (A44)$$

With that we obtain

$$A_{sum}(x,t) = 2 \cdot (A_o \cdot (\cos \delta/2) \cdot (\sin 2\pi) \cdot (x/\lambda - v \cdot t + \delta/2)) \quad (A45)$$

or

$$A_{sum}(x,t) = A_{sum,o} \sin 2\pi \ (x/\lambda - v \ t + \delta/2) \quad (A46)$$

with

$$A_{sum,o} = 2 \cdot A_o \cdot \cos \delta/2. \quad (A47)$$

Equation A47 describes a wave with the same properties as the both original waves, except that it is shifted in phase by $\delta/2$, i.e. halfway between the former. But look at the amplitude: when the both original waves are in phase ($\delta=0$) then $A_{sum,o}=2A_o$, i.e. the amplitudes just add up (since cos 0=1) as one might have expected. When they are, however, shifted by a half wavelength ($\delta=\pi$) then the amplitude is zero (since cos $\pi/2=0$) for all times. Amplitudes cannot be measured, but their squares can. They are the intensities of the waves. We will come back to this later. Here we note that two waves can totally cancel each other. This is remarkable since two waves, both carrying energy and momentum, add up to nothing – the energy appears to be going to nowhere.

For the purposes of this book two other aspects are interesting:

- If an object is invisible, since it is transparent but induces a phase shift in light-waves, it can be made visible by overlaying an unshifted wave, since interference then causes differences in intensity. This fact has been used in phase contrast microscopy (Section 1.3.1)
- If it is known how the amplitudes of two waves in phase should add up one can calculate the phase shift induced by an object in the path of one wave by measuring the intensity of the sum wave. This is used for the very precise localization of particles in optical tweezers as indicated in Section 2.6.5.

## A4.4 Standing waves and modes

Assume now that a wave is spatially confined by two mirrors. It will hit the mirror, be reflected, hit the other mirror, be reflected and so on. The wave and the reflected wave will add up. Formally the two waves are described by

$$A(x,t) = A_o \cdot (\sin 2\pi) \cdot (x/\lambda - v \cdot t) \quad (A48)$$

and

$$A(x,t) = A_o \cdot (\sin 2\pi) \cdot (x/\lambda + v \cdot t). \quad (A49)$$

With the same type of calculus as above, using the same formula from trigonometry, one obtains a totally different type of result:

$$A_{sum}(x,t) = A_{sum,o} \cdot (\cos 2\pi) \cdot v \quad (A50)$$

this is no longer a travelling wave, since the argument of the cosine no longer contains the position x. Instead, the amplitude is dependent on position

$$A_{sum,o} = 2 \cdot (A_o \cdot (\sin 2\pi) \cdot x/\lambda) \quad (A51)$$

For example, at x=0 and for all half integer multiples of $\lambda$ the amplitude is zero at all times, since the sine is zero at these values. What we have found is a standing wave with nodes and antinodes. However, so far we have omitted an important fact: this standing wave only evolves when the distance l between the two mirrors and the wavelength are related by

$$\lambda = 2 \cdot l/n \quad n = 1, 2, 3,\ldots\ldots \quad (A52)$$

i.e. when the waves fully fit in between the two mirrors. This is the resonance condition for the wave in a two-mirror system, i.e. the optical resonator of a laser (Section 1.2.5). It is observed when half a wave fits between the mirrors, but also when two, three four and so on half wavelengths fit. The different forms of standing waves are called "modes". Usually a resonator supports standing waves satisfying the resonance condition for n=1. Since this is the longest possible wavelength which requires a minimum of energy to cause resonance, this "ground mode" is highly favored. However, when a large amount of energy is available, higher modes can also have substantial intensity. In some materials part of the ground mode may then switch into a higher mode. Everybody has probably heard this when a pipe is blown with too much effort: then a very high tone is produced, corresponding to the half wavelength (double frequency, octave) or even higher "harmonics". A process similar to this is used in laser systems for frequency doubling, tripling etc. (Section 1.2.6).

# A5 Absorption, scattering and fluorescence

## A5.1 Absorption and scattering make objects visible and allow work to be done on them

Micromanipulation by light is a novel type of microscopy. An object is first visualized at low light intensities and then light of high power density is used to work on it.

But what does "visualizing" mean? There are several basic mechanisms which can be exploited to visualize microscopic objects. Somehow light coming from the object has to be imaged onto the retina of the observer's eye, where the optical signal is converted into an electrical signal and further transmitted to the brain. The light may be produced by the object itself. A star in the sky is seen due to the light it had emitted as the final result of events powered by a nuclear reaction. In the microscope, objects may be caused to emit light as a consequence of a chemical reaction (chemoluminescence). Also, certain dyes can be induced to emit visible light by illuminating them with invisible light or with light of an other color (fluorescence). In conclusion, an object can be imaged by the light it emits.

But most events we see in everyday life and in most forms of microscopy do not rely on emission but on several types of reflection or light scattering. An object is illuminated by an external light source. Light of the same wavelength is finally used by the eye for detection. For example, when a white wall is illuminated by a white light source (such as the sun) it will scatter all colors. The direction of the scattered light cannot be predicted. The light is dispersed. In contrast, light from a mirror is reflected rather than scattered, i.e. the direction of light falling onto the surface and the direction of the light leaving it are highly correlated. Therefore the spatial relationship of all details of the object are preserved and one can really recognize an image of it. In the microscope, reflection can be a mechanism to image objects.

A further basic mechanism is absorption. Absorption of red components of sunlight (which is a mixture of all colors) and scattering of other colors is responsible for the fact that the leaves of plants appear green. Correspondingly, blood absorbs blue and green and therefore appears red. When an object absorbs many colors it appears black and may thus be visualized by light missing from the illumination. Absorption is also the first step in generating fluorescence. Thus

*Images of objects are often generated by absorbed or reflected light.*
*Colors are generated by absorption of components of white light.*

Absorption, scattering and reflection are also relevant when high light intensities are used to work on microscopic objects. Since the absorbed light energy may be converted into heat, the object may be destroyed. This is the basic process underlying the microbeam technique. When light of high intensity is scattered or reflected, it will exert considerable forces on the scattering object. This is the basic process underlying optical tweezers.

Strictly speaking, light is not absorbed or scattered by the objects but by their atoms or molecules. The following discussion concerns atoms, but applies equally well for molecules. An atom can exist in different energy states. When it is left alone for a sufficiently long time it will be in a state of minimum energy, its ground state. Then, all electrons are as close to the nucleus as the balance of attracting and repelling forces allows. One of many possible states of higher energy of this atom would be its ion, a state where at least one electron is missing. In order to ionize an atom one has provide energy. In turn, when an ion catches an electron to become an atom again, energy is released. This can be registered by an increase in temperature or occasionally, by emission of light.

Ionization is a quite dramatic modification of an atom. A more gentle change is to increase the average distance of the outermost electron from the nucleus. This process also requires energy, just as energy is required for an aircraft to increase its distance from the Earth's center when it gains height. Since in an atom the space is limited it acts as a resonator. In Appendix A4.4 it was shown that in a resonator standing waves are expected. Each mode corresponds to a well-defined amount of energy. A transition from, for example the mode of lowest energy (the ground state) to a mode of higher energy (an excited state) requires a well-defined amount of energy. The atom can exist in the excited state for a few nanoseconds. Then it will often emit light, it will fluoresce.

Many types of energy sources may drive the excitation, for example, heat (this is why a burning flame or hot metal emit light), an electric current (as, for example, in light tubes) or even sound. A very precise and efficient energy source for such a transition is light impinging on the atom, but only when it has a frequency for which $E=h\cdot v$ approximately fits the energy difference between ground state and excited state. Then this portion of energy is removed from the light wave; it is absorbed, and the atom is excited. If the wavelength does not fit, i.e. if a suitable energy portion cannot be exchanged, no absorption occurs.

This description of the absorption process implies that the atom determines the frequency and thus the wavelength of light which can interact, and also the energy size of the quantum which is exchanged. It never occurs that light with the incorrect wavelength imprints its own properties onto the atom. In this sense, absorption of light by an atom means removing a quantum of energy (a photon) from light passing along it.

## A5.2 Absorption and emission in a two-state atom

As indicated, in an atom many energy states are possible. Studying these states is the subject of spectroscopy. For the purposes of this book we need only up to four states, and for the time being we can restrict ourselves to two states. Thus, for the following discussion it is assumed that the atom has only a ground state, "a", and one excited state "b". Without external stimuli (i.e. in thermal equilibrium at a given temperature) in an ensemble of atoms $n_a$ atoms are in the ground state and $n_b$ atoms are in the excited state. Three different processes between a and b may be powered by the interaction with light:

1. Light of suitable wavelength can be absorbed by an atom which is in the ground state. The atom is then electronically excited.
   This process is quantified by a rate constant $B_{ab}$.
2. The excited atom will not remain in the excited state forever. After some time it will return to the ground state, often by re-emission of light. For an individual atom one cannot predict how long it will take before this process, called

"spontaneous emission", occurs. For a large number of atoms or molecules of the same type one can find an average value, which is called the lifetime of the excited state.

This process is quantified by a rate constant $A_{ba}$.

3. Re-emission can also be stimulated by light of a wavelength similar to that of the light to be emitted. This process is called "stimulated emission". This process is quantified by the rate constant $B_{ba}$.

Strictly speaking, absorption is also a stimulated process, since it is dependent on $I(l)$, the intensity of the incoming light. The rates of the two stimulated processes can be calculated as

$$\text{Rate}_{abs} = n_a \cdot B_{ab} \cdot I(\lambda) \quad (A53)$$

and

$$\text{Rate}_{stim.emiss.} = n_b \cdot B_{ba} \cdot I(\lambda). \quad (A54)$$

In contrast to the two stimulated processes spontaneous emission is independent of any incoming light. The rate constant $A_{ba}$ is dependent on the dipole strength $D_{ba}$, a quantity which describes how strongly the two states a and b are coupled to each other. In order to calculate $D_{ba}$ detailed quantum mechanical calculation is required.

The reciprocal of the rate constant for spontaneous emission is called the natural lifetime of the state b. Thus:

$$1/\tau = A_{ba} = \text{const} \cdot \lambda^{-3} \cdot D_{ab}. \quad (A55)$$

Since this rate inversely depends on the third power of the wavelength it is, for example, by a factor of 8 larger at the UV wavelength of 300 nm than in the red at 600 nm. In other words, spontaneous emission is very high (or the lifetime of the corresponding state is low), when the result is UV light and lower by almost an order of magnitude when red light is emitted.

## A5.3 The Lambert Beer law

For many substances the calculation of the (spontaneous) absorption is difficult since a number of quantum mechanical details are required. Such information is often not available, even for quite simple materials which may serve as laser media. For biological molecules, it is even more difficult to calculate absorption properties. Therefore, most data are experimentally determined using the Lambert Beer law, which assumes the intensity of light falling on a thin layer of a material with the thickness dx is reduced by absorption by the fraction dI / I. In many cases, the absorbing layer is a solution of molecules having the concentration c. The material properties can then be described by the material factor $\varepsilon$, the molar extinction coefficient and the absorption can be described formally as

$$dI/I = \varepsilon \cdot c \cdot dx \quad \text{(A56)}$$

Note that the symbol $\varepsilon$ has been used as dielectric constant in other parts of the book. Since this double use is also the case in the literature and since the danger of mixing the two up is small, this inconvenience may not be too serious. Equation A56 is a simple differential equation which often occurs in nature. Prominent cases where it holds are radioactive decay and fluorescence decay. The quantities dx and dI are "differentials" indicating that the equation is strictly valid only for infinitesimally small layer thickness dx and infinitesimally small intensity losses dI. According to simple mathematical laws equation A56 can be integrated

$$\ln I(x)/I_0 = \varepsilon \cdot c \cdot x \quad \text{(A57)}$$

where the left side is a natural logarithm.

Applying the exponential function exp on both sides and using the fact that for any function

$$\exp \ln Y = Y, \quad \text{(A58)}$$

one obtains

$$I(x)/I_0 = \exp(-\varepsilon \cdot c \cdot x) \quad \text{(A59)}$$

or

$$I(x) = I_0 \cdot \exp(-\varepsilon \cdot c \cdot x) \quad (A60)$$

When the intensities in front and after a cuvette of thickness x containing a solution with concentration c of a molecule are measured, the molar absorption coefficient can be calculated by equation A60. In turn, once the molar absorption coefficient is known, one can calculate its concentration in an unknown solution.

The molar absorption coefficient is a macroscopic quantity. Since it is expressed in liter per mole and cm, one can calculate from it directly the corresponding term for atomar or molecular absorption, since $1 \, mol = 6 \cdot 10^{23}$ molecules. For a molecule with for example a molar absorption coefficient of 1000 liter mol$^{-1}$cm$^{-1}$ the calculation is as follows:

$$\varepsilon = 1000 \, liter \cdot mol^{-1} \cdot cm^{-1}$$

$$\varepsilon = 1000 \, liter \cdot 1/6 \cdot 10^{-23} \, molecules \cdot cm^{-1}$$

$$\varepsilon = 1/6 \cdot 10^{-16} \, cm^2 \quad (A61)$$

This molecular quantity now gets the symbol $a_1$, has the dimension of an area and is called the molecular or atomar "absorption cross section". Equation A56 now becomes

$$k = \alpha_1 \cdot I \quad (A62)$$

where k is a rate constant, the number of absorbed photons per incident photon and per second when I is given in photons per cm$^2$ and per second.

## A5.4 Two- and three-photon absorption

At sufficiently high intensities, an atom or molecule can absorb two, three or more light quanta simultaneously. Since the energy gap in an atom is given (see, for example, Fig. A11), only two quanta with half the energy (the double wavelength) of the gap or three quanta with a third of this energy can be absorbed. The equations corresponding to equation are:

$$k = \alpha_2 \cdot I^2 \quad (A63)$$

$$k = \alpha_3 \cdot I^3 \quad (A64)$$

For four-, five- ... photon processes the equations have to be modified correspondingly. However, when more than a few light quanta cooperate, the macroscopic treatment as it was chosen in the main text (Sections 2.1 through 2.3) is adequate and more convenient. Box A9 gives, for a few dye molecules, $\alpha_1$, $\alpha_2$ and $\alpha_3$ at selected wavelengths. By using such cross sections and equations A62 through A64, one can see that, in order to get a similar number of absorptions per molecule, a $10^4$- to $10^5$-fold higher intensity is required for the two- and three-photon effect than for one-photon effect. At the light intensities achieved with laser microbeams and also with optical tweezers, multiphoton processes are possible.

### Box A9: Molecular absorption cross sections for dye molecules

| Cross section | | $10^{-16}$ cm$^2$ | $10^{-49}$ cm$^4$s | $10^{-83}$ cm$^6$s$^2$ |
|---|---|---|---|---|
| Wavelength | | 335–362 nm | 700 nm | 1000 nm |
| DAPI | 345 nm | 1.3 | 0.016 | 0.25 |
| Dansyl | 336 nm | 0.17 | 0.1 | 0.3 |
| Fura + Ca | 335 nm | 1.2 | 1.2 | 30 |
| Fura | 362 nm | 1.0 | 1.1 | 20 |
| Indo + Ca | 340 nm | 1.3 | 0.15 | 6 |
| Indo free | 345 nm | 1.3 | 0.35 | 2 |
| APSS | at 800nm | | 380 | |
| ASPT | at 1064nm | | 1200 | |

data from: C.X. Warren Zippel, J.B. Shear, R.M. Williams, W.W. Webb (1996) Proc. Natl. Acad. Sci. 10763-10768, Multiphoton fluorescence excitation: New spectral windows for biological nonlinear microscopy and (APSS, ASPT); P.C. Cheng, S.J. Pan, A. Shih, K.S. Kim, W.S. Liou, M.S. Park (1998) J. Mic. 189.3, 199-212, Highly efficient upconverters for multiphoton fluorescence microcopy.

## A5.5 Rayleigh scattering

Scattering is the second basic process underlying micromanipulation by light. It will ultimately determine the force which light is exerting on matter. The theoretical formalism to calculate scattering depends on the ratio of the wavelength of scattered light to the size of the scatterer. The best understood situation is given for small molecules, i.e. for a situation where the wavelength is much larger than the scattering object. This is the regime of Rayleigh scattering.

The theory of Rayleigh scattering uses the fact that the particles are dipoles. A statical dipole consists of two opposite charges. If these are oscillating against each other it is a dynamic dipole. The alternating electric field strength of a light wave can induce such dynamic dipoles in molecules of dielectric material. Like microscopic antenna, the latter emit an electromagnetic wave into selected directions of space. The quantitative value of the light power W involved in this process follows from antenna theory:

$$W = \omega^4 \cdot D^2 / 6\pi \cdot \varepsilon_0 \cdot c^3 \quad (A61)$$

$$\omega = 2\pi \cdot v = 2\pi \cdot c / \lambda \quad (A62)$$

where D is the dipole moment and all other quantities as defined above. D can be correlated with the polarizability $\alpha$ by

$$D = \alpha \cdot E. \quad (A63)$$

Combining equations A61 to A63 allows expressing W in terms of the light intensity I and the polarizability $\alpha$

$$W = I \cdot (8\pi^3 / 3\varepsilon_0) \cdot \alpha^2 \quad (A64)$$

The polarizability $\alpha$ can be related to the dielectricity constants $\varepsilon_0$ of the vacuum and e of the scattering material via a relationship which is called the Clausius Masotti relationship

$$\alpha = 3\varepsilon_0 \cdot (\varepsilon-1)/((\varepsilon+2) \cdot V) \quad (A65)$$

where V is the volume of one scattering molecule. Combining equations A64 and A65 and using the fact that

$$V = 4/3r^3\pi \quad (A66)$$

and that for non magnetic particles $\varepsilon = n^2$ (with n = refractive index of the particle) one obtains

$$W = I \cdot (128\pi^5 r^6/3\lambda^4) \cdot ((n^2-1)/(n^2+2))^2 \quad (A67)$$

This equation was the basis for the discussion in Box 25 of Section 2.4.3.

## A5.6 The detailed two energy state diagram of fluorescence

As was mentioned in the previous chapter, the lifetime of an excited state is given by the dipole strength of a pair of energy states. If this is very large, its lifetime is short (picoseconds or below) and one speaks of a virtual energy state. When such a short-living virtual state is involved, one does not speak of absorption and emission but of scattering. Since the scattering molecule does not move or rotate significantly during the short time of excitation, the angular distribution of the scattered light is still related to the direction of the incoming light. The situation changes when the lifetime of a state approaches the nanosecond range. Then light is emitted isotropically into all directions of space. This is fluorescence. The energy states are said to be real. By now it is not clear where the borderline between scattering and fluorescence has to be set. Thus, in the lifetime range between pico- and nanoseconds the notation is not definitely clear. In spite of this there is a clear way to distinguish between fluorescence and most types of scattering. Most scattering processes are elastic, i.e. only the direction of the light but not the wavelength changes. Others are inelastic in a way that, at each wavelength the energy difference between exciting and scattered light is the same.

On the contrary, fluorescence emission occurs at fixed higher wavelengths (further in the red region) when it is excited by different wavelengths further in the blue. Only the fluorescence intensity changes. The basic mechanism is not evident from Appendix A5 which was too simple. We did not consider that in addition to electronic excitation from the gound state to the first excited state, there can also occur vibrational and rotational excitation. Chemical bonds in molecules vibrate. They can do this with various frequencies which can be calculated from quantum mechanics. The result is that the ground state as well as the electronically excited state are not as well defined as suggested by the simple two state model. There are bundles of states rather than single states. The former are higher than the pure electronic states. Fig. A11 shows a correspondingly extended diagram.

Therefore, the excitation can go from a higher state to a variety of rotational and vibrational states above the corresponding electronic states. For absorption, one consequence is that instead of a sharp absorption line, particularly in biological molecules in aqueous solutions, a broad absorption band is observed. For emission this means that it occurs at longer wavelengths (smaller energies), since the vibrational excitation first relaxes within picoseconds, producing heat. After nanoseconds, light is emitted. Since the transition in most cases ends in a vibrationally excited state of the bundle of ground states, the energy difference is again smaller than in the simple two-state model and therefore shifted to red wavelengths. Since these states relax very fast while the lowest vibrational state has a lifetime of several nanoseconds, the vibration first relaxes. This energy is dissipated as heat. It stays in the lowest vibrational state of the first excited state for the duration of a fluorescence lifetime. Only then does the molecule emit light.

## A5.7 Fluorescence and phosphorescence lifetimes as a basis for explaining laser action

Above, the lifetimes of energy levels were mentioned, but only used as the inverse of decay rate constants. In fluorescence spectroscopy these lifetimes are explicitly measured since, in addition they give information about to the spectra. The lifetime of an energy level does not mean that in an ensemble of atoms or molecules each one remains excited for exactly the lifetime. Spontaneous emission refers rather to a statistical process. One excited state may spontaneosly emit a photon immediately after it has been excited. Others may rest very long in the excited state. Only when the time between excitation and spontaneous emission of many molecules is measured can one determine the lifetime of the excited state. There are several ways to measure lifetimes. Conceptually the most simple, though not the most economic, way is to excite a sample of molecules with a weak short light pulse, formerly

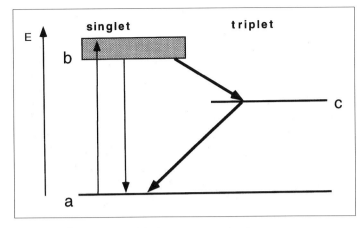

**Fig. A11:** *Three-state model of an atom or molecule.*

by a flash lamp, today almost exclusively with lasers. Many atoms will be excited. The first photon which will be re-emitted is detected by a photomultiplier. After repeating this process many times, the number of results with a given time difference between excitation and emission, corrected by time differences solely caused by the apparatus, is plotted logarithmically versus the time difference. Fig. A12 gives such a result for the amino acid tryptophan.

The result is a straight line, representing an exponential decay, similarly as with the radioactive decay of material. The lifetime $\tau$ is the decay time after which the number of events has decreased to 1/e (e=2.71) of the value at time zero. Occasionally, instead of the lifetime the time after which the number of events has decreased to 50% of the original value, $T_{1/2}$, is used. The relationship between both is

$$T_{1/2} = 0.693 \cdot \tau. \quad (A68)$$

Examples of such monoexponential decays are rarely observed. Usually the plots as in Fig. A12 are curved. Occasionally the reason for such a multiexponential decay is that the the fluorescing part of a molecule, for example the tyrosine in a protein, occurs in different physicochemical microenvironments, which all exert different influences over the lifetime. Such structural variants can sometimes be confirmed by nuclear magnetic resonance experiments or fluorescence quenching studies.

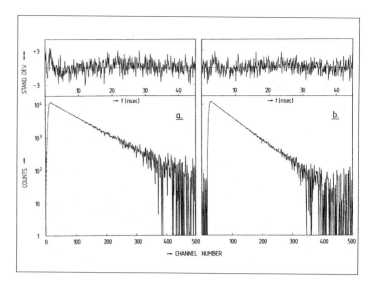

**Fig. A12:** *Fluorescence decay curve for tryptophan.*

The natural lifetimes of energy levels are in the order of 20-30 ns, the true lifetimes are smaller due to a plethora of processes which can reduce them. Quite often, however, lifetimes of microseconds up to seconds are observed. This is then dubbed phosphorescence and can be observed as a long lasting afterglow of objects such as the clock-face of a watch. At a first glance, phosphorescence seems to differ from fluorescence only by the lifetime of its excited energy state but the physical basis is conceptually different and it is the basics for the laser process.

Many dye molecules are so complex that they have, in addition to their main electronically excited state level, at least one further level. Often this is a triplet state. Such states are very important for spectroscopy. For the purposes of this book it is sufficient to know that transitions between the energy states described so far (which are dubbed singlet states) and triplet states are forbidden. As in real life, that does not prevent molecules from supporting such transitions, though with much lower probability than singlet-singlet transition. Thus it is difficult but not impossible for a molecule to come into a triplet state by a process called "intersystem crossing". The emission of a photon by transition of the atom or molecule from a triplet state to the ground state (which is a singlet state) is forbidden as well. The consequence is that the triplet state has a very long lifetime and emits a low number of photons per time unit. Therefore, phosphorescence is not very suitable for highly sensitive detection of molecules, but it is interesting when long-term processes are required, as is the case, for example, with lasers.

# Index